Teeth in Your Mouth

Pathologist's foray into dental hygiene

Izak Dimenstein

Teeth in Your Mouth

Pathologist's foray into personal dental hygiene

Izak B. Dimenstein, MD, PhD, HT (ASCP)

Disclaimer

The author disclaims any liability for any medical damage concerning using any information presented in this book.

Acknowledgment

Thanks to Elena, Simon, and Eugene Dimenstein for editorial and technical support in the publication of this book.

Table of Contents

Preface

Hygiea was assigned by her father, the god of medicine, Asclepius, to be in charge of health, cleanliness, and sanitation. In contrast to her sister, the lightheaded Panacea, who became synonymous with unachievable universal remedies, Hygiea was a no-nonce woman who required certain actions from people to keep their bodies in check, including their teeth. She didn't leave behind any specifics. People have written a great deal of literature on her behalf. Perhaps this current book contributes to that literature.

This book is about the care of teeth, which are intentionally placed first in the title. Of course, teeth are located in the mouth. Where they dwell cannot be ignored, but the book emphasizes teeth. Dental or oral hygiene is the personal maintenance of teeth and gums. It is related to, but different from, dental hygienists' service as part of professional dentistry.

Many books have been written about this subject. For example, *Understanding Your Teeth and Mouth* by David and Alyson Wray or *Holistic Dental Care: The Complete Guide to Healthy Teeth and Gums* by Nadine Artemis, *Dr. Ben's Dental Notebook: A Collection of Dental Illustrations, Handouts and Diagrams* by Dr. Ben Magleby are excellent publications with similar titles. *The Great Tooth Deception* by Heither Hygienist's book is interesting by challenging the entire dental care enterprise isn't of my book's scope.

The published in 2022 *book If Your Mouth Could Talk: An In-Depth Guide to Oral Health and Its Impact on Your Entire Life*, written by renowned orthodontist and dentofacial orthopedist Dr. Kami Hoss, is interesting and well designed. The annotation on Amazon presents it as *USA TODAY* and *Wall Street Journal* bestseller. Dr. Hoss propagates a holistic approach to "oral health" as the balance of mouth microbes (microbiome), "which can wreak havoc or support wellness, and health growth and development of the structures of the mouth, which result in good airways and well-formed faces." Although the book is addressing predominately children health, the author's meaning of "overall heals" encompass" physical health, social well-being, mental health, success in life, and longevity." This conceptual book is not about brushing and flossing or other standard dental hygiene standard procedures recommended in the dentist office.

I am quoting this book because the author's, a practicing professional in the field, main premises of biological approach of oral health presented in coherent   persuasive way, reflects also my main premises of evolutionary approach to teeth dwelling in the mouth, as a result of the microbiota evolutionary development.

My book is also conceptual. However, my current book differs in terms of my approaches to the subject and the format in which I will present the material. In contrast to Dr. Hoss's book, I am concentrating on the details of dental hygiene procedure, just brushing, flossing, and rinsing.

I'm bringing my pathology practitioner vision to dental hygiene's well-established practices while following the commonly accepted principles. Pathology, as a part of medicine, takes a broad, holistic approach to biological processes in the human body. The pathophysiology branch tends to have experimental proof of assumptions. Anatomic pathology uses autopsy and morphology studies, including histology, to visualize data for interpretation.

It would be reasonable to present my background, which incorporates medical science (MD), general biology as an experimental immunologist in a pathophysiology Ph.D. program, and experience as an anatomic pathology practitioner, having performed thousands of autopsies. I've spent many years as a grossing technologist in the surgical pathology histology laboratory, where methodology details are paramount in developing the final product—a micro slide for the pathologist's diagnosis. Scrupulous attention to detail was the leading driver in writing this personal dental hygiene book.

The maxim states: "There is nothing as practical as a good theory." This is why this book contains theoretical considerations. They are one of the book's goals to bring science and rationality into commonly accepted practices.

While concentrating on details, I explain WHY the recommended action is taken. Certain situations in everyday life often require people to accommodate the recommended standard routine. The main actions will be followed if a person understands the procedure's aim.

The book is designed in my workshop PowerPoint style of writing professional books with diagrams and illustrations. This writing style adapts to a modern person's TV and now video clip way of consuming information, which aligns with the infographic summarization of important points of the topic.

I do not expect this book to be read from cover to cover. The reader can explore the areas of most interest. In this regard, one can start by reading my practical suggestions in the *Methods and Tools* part and later go to the entries in the *General and Specials* parts. Often boring and sometimes inevitably repetitious, both parts provide necessary background information for my recommendations.

I published *Everyday Dental Care* book where "theoretical" part of the current book is omitted. Instead, I placed some examples of current brands of paste and mouthwash with photos of ingredients on the labels. This might help to choose preferred items .at home instead of the stores shelfs. I do not advertise any of them. My goal is only information without personal bias.

Entries that would not fit the main parts of the book are placed in the *Appendices*. Some of them are mostly assumptions but might interest a curious reader. Bridges, and now implants, require strict adherence to the principles of personal dental hygiene (see *Remarks on Dental Bridges' Longevity* in the *Appendices*). Moreover, dental construction becomes more vulnerable with age and less resistant to the challenges of modern food consumption.

This book is not a scholar study. Few books or other published materials are used as references. I am offering my views and assumptions as my pathologist's foray into dental hygiene.

The book's intention is a modest one. I want to find my informational space between academic research publications, popular books and the fragmented sources disseminated on the internet, such as Google Search, Wikipedia articles, and Artificial Intelligence (AI) overviews.

This is friendly talk with people who care for their teeth—the wonderful device presented to humans by nature. People who have lost some parts of this device can join this conversation. I would be glad if this book added additional information to what is already known or even changed some people's views of well-established knowledge.

General Part

The anatomic and physiological descriptions in this book provide minimal data related to understanding individual dental hygiene actions or inactions. Some descriptions are short, while others are disproportionally long. Many theoretical considerations might be boring and look superfluous, but without them, I cannot present my vision of dental hygiene practice, my suggestions, and my recommendations.

A short excursion into the origins of teeth reminds us that they are part of human evolution. This view is common knowledge.

Interestingly by themselves, data of teeth ancestry are presented to underline that our dental hygiene actions should take into account that we are dealing with established teeth and the mouth's biological structure from millions of years ago. Any intrusion into this complicated environment should be done with caution.

Teeth remote ancestry

Where do human teeth come from? I compiled the short answer to this question from many sources. The main one is *Human Anatomy* by M. Prives et al., 1984, a textbook for medical schools.

Evolutionary, teeth are derived from scales of fish that grow along the edge of the jaws but acquire new functions. Since teeth wear away, they are shed and replaced by new ones. This occurs repeatedly many times in lover vertebrates and only twice in man, as deciduous and permanent teeth.

The shark's structure contains the most important parts of the tooth, enamel, and dentin. During evolution, two parts became distinguishable in the teeth of reptiles: the root, which is lodged in the jaws' alveoli, and the external part, the crown.

The diversity of food eaten by terrestrial animals (*terra*-earth in Latin) determined the development of their masticatory apparatus and teeth specialization. As a consequence, in distinction from the monotypic conic teeth of fish, which serve only for the retention of food, the teeth of mammals acquired different shapes adapted to grasping and treating various types of food, namely tearing (the canine teeth), cutting (the incisor teeth), crushing (the premolar teeth), and grinding (the molar teeth).

People, being able to eat both plants and meat (omnivorous), have preserved all these teeth. Since the function of grasping changed from the jaws to the hands, the jaws became different, and the teeth became smaller. The number of teeth in the New World monkeys is 36 (2 1 3 3), and in the Old-World monkeys, 32 (2 1 2 3). In man, the development of the third molar (the 'wisdom tooth') is delayed, reflecting the teeth' tendency to regression. A toothless man has been described as a case of anomaly.

The teeth were the first hard structures in the body of ancient vertebrates, developing before the other parts of the skeleton. Paleontologists established that vertebrates originated in the Paleozoic era from the discovery of teeth, the only remnants of that time. Since the shape of teeth corresponds to the type of nutrition and the mode of life, paleontologists recognize the fossils of animals and human beings by teeth.

Evolutionary teeth were designed for certain life conditions until the pressure of natural selection ended almost 40,000 years ago. At that time, some rare individuals reached old age. Changes to people's longevity, lifestyle, and nutrition should be considered in relation to the current care of teeth while keeping in mind evolutionary ancestry.

Anatomy

Anatomy and physiology of teeth and mouth data relate only to the book's subject. . I would call them as functional anatomy. Namely, prophylactic teeth care. For the same reason completely omitted the deciduous (milk) teeth development, their time of eruption, and changes for permanent teeth.

 Only anatomical terms related to dental hygiene procedures are used. All of them will be mentioned in the Special Part.

Residency in the mouth

A tooth is an ossified papillae of the jaw's mucous membrane for the mechanical treatment of food.

The teeth are located in the alveolar processes of the maxilla (upper teeth) and mandible (lower teeth) bones. They are fitted into the jaws. Each row consists of 16 teeth arranged as a dental arch.

The tissue covering the alveolar processes is called the gums (gingivae). The mucous membrane is closely joined to the bone (periosteum) here using fibrous tissue (periodontium); the gingival tissue is rich in blood vessels and bleeds relatively easily but is poor in nerves. The grooved depression between the tooth and the free margin of the gum is called the gingival pocket.

The tooth, the periodontium, the alveolar wall, and the gingiva compose the **tooth organ**.

32 teeth team

There are four types of teeth. Their function is different. **Incisors**, four on each jaw, have a crown shaped like a cutting chisel; they cut food to the needed size. The crown of the upper incisors is twice the width of the lower incisors.

Canines two of each jaw. They acquired a well-developed crown serving for crushing and grinding food while maintaining the ancient function of the tooth, i.e., cutting and tearing food.

Premolars four from each side. Presence on the masticating surface of the crown of two masticating or occlusion eminences, or cusps (photo below). This shape of the crowns enables the premolars to grind the food into small fragments.

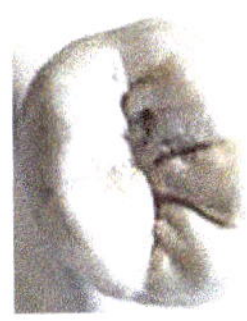 Molar eminences, or cusps.

Molars six from on each Jaw. They are smaller from front to back. The first molar is the largest. The third is the smallest.

The latter erupts late and is called the wisdom tooth (dens sapiential). The shape of the crown, more or less square with three or more cusps, determines the function of the molars—they grind food. The cusps will be mentioned many times in the toothbrushing section. They need special treatment during brushing due to their irregular form, which could trap food remnants.

Tooth structure

Each tooth (*dens* in Latin) consists of a crown, a neck, and a root. The gum embraces the neck (a slightly narrowed part of the tooth), while the root sits in the dental alveolus. A small opening in the apex is seen even with the naked eye.

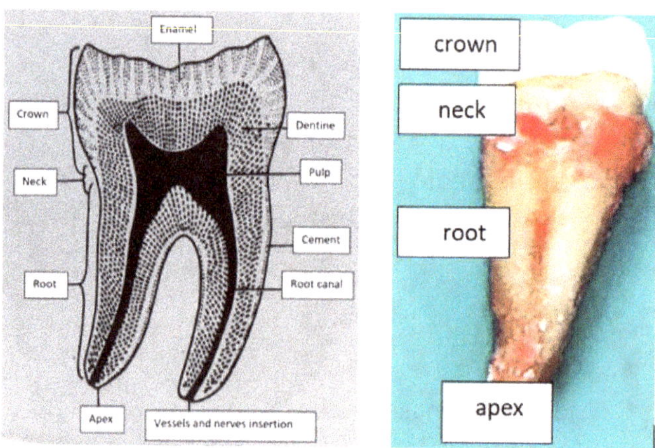

Four parts are distinguished: the crown, the widest part, the root part, and the narrowed part of the cavity called the root canal. The canal opens at the apex. The tooth root fuses tightly with the surface of the tooth alveolar bone of the jaws using the alveolar periodontium. Vessels and nerves enter the tooth through the opening in the apex.

Periodontal ligament

A tooth is situated in the jaw bone but does not directly touch the bone. It is held in the socket by the periodontal ligament, commonly abbreviated as the PDL, which is only found between the root part of the tooth and the adjacent bone. This structure requires a more detailed presentation related to prophylactic dental care.

The periodontal ligament (PDL) is a group of specialized connective tissue fibers of various collagen types. It has a highly narrow and complex neurovascular component—the ligament inserts into the root cementum from one side and onto the alveolar bone on the other. Although called a ligament, PDL is unlike ligaments surrounding an articulating joint. PDL is what holds teeth in place. Its width -0.15-0.38 mm; the thinnest portion is around the middle third of the root. The interdental papillae, as part of the gingiva, prevent food impaction.

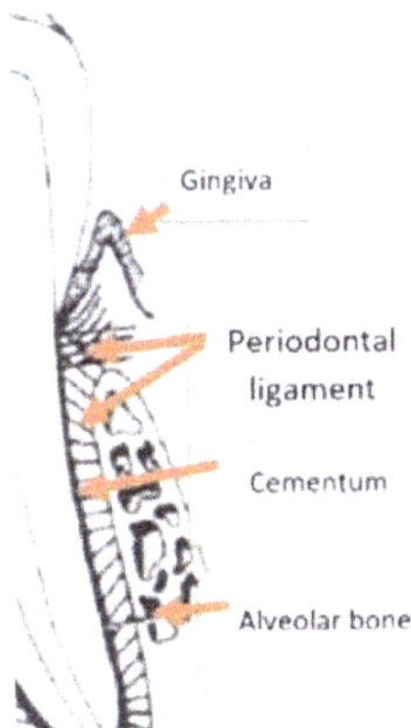

Periodontal ligament (PDL).

This complex tissue allows the tooth to function under the chewing load and absorb excess pressure from clenching and grinding. This system is designed to withstand and exert forces in a vertical vector (chewing). The teeth are weakest in shear forces.

PDL is involved in tooth movement to adjust to the food's firmness. Otherwise, the tooth would be prone to crashes. In other words, the tooth is held in the socket by the periodontal ligament, which acts as a shock absorber. Along with the enamel, the periodontal ligament is like a car suspension. Challenging the car suspension regularly is not the best driving habit.

The periodontal ligament also allows the tooth to adapt to forces from tooth grinding (bruxism) or other jaw-clenching habits. The ligament can enlarge and allow the tooth to become loose. Once the excessive forces on the tooth are reduced, the PDL will heal, and tooth mobility will decrease.

The Special Part will discuss the significance of maintaining PDL integrity in periodontal health.

Bite

When the upper and lower teeth come in contact (occlusion), the upper incisors overlap and partially cover the lower incisors. This occurs because the maxillary dental arch is slightly larger than the mandibular one. There is no full congruence between low and upper teeth: each tooth comes not with one but two teeth from another side. This is a concern for the consequences of tooth extraction.

Two variants of normal bite (occlusion) are distinguished according to relationships between upper front teeth and lower front teeth. The first is called a scissor-like bite. It is encountered in most individuals 80%. In this type of occlusion, the upper teeth' cutting edges overlap the lower teeth' cutting edges.

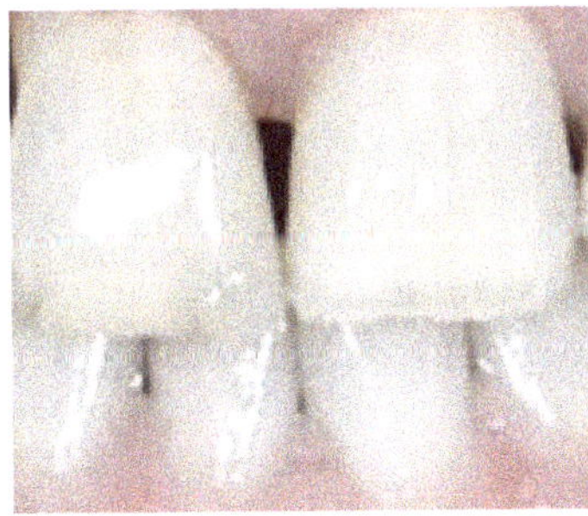

Scissor-like bite

The second variant is called tongue-like bite. In this type of bite, the cutting edges of the upper anterior teeth meet the cutting edges of the lower anterior teeth. It mainly occurs in childhood (in attrition of the teeth) and in the elderly.

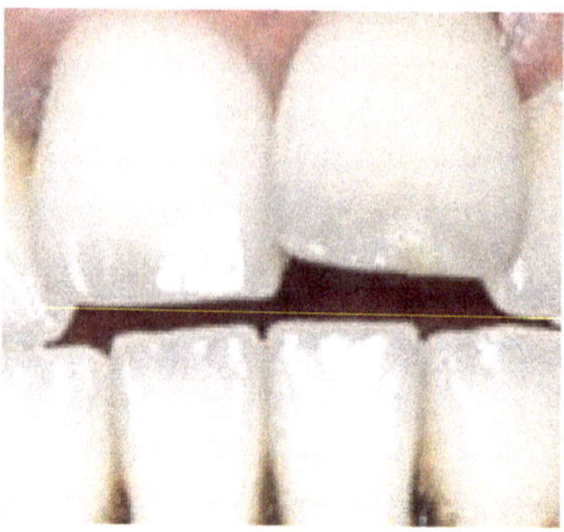

Tongue-like bite

There is no significant difference in toothbrushing, although the scissor-like bite requires a more open mouth during brushing. It is more critical in teeth whitening.

Pathologic bites, Abnormal numbers of teeth, and the position and shape of crowns or roots are outside the scope of this book. However, they can bring some particularities in individual dental hygiene techniques, for example, during flossing.

Tongue

The tongue is a significant part of the mouth anatomy that plays a role in dental hygiene. The tongue " rants" the middle and upper floors of the mouth. On the upper floor, closer to the pharynx, called the root or the back, multiple relatively large papillae hide different microorganisms. In this "forest," many microorganisms can be lost because they are not fleshed out by saliva, which tends to be on the lower floor of the mouth.

 Four areas should be distinguished for dental hygiene procedures. The main 2/3 space is for facing the teeth/mouth part. At the tip is a delicate place with tactile and taste receptors. Numerous filiform and conical papillae are located here. This area hosts different kinds of microorganisms, including bad breath bacteria.

Visible as a groove, the median sulcus can also hide excesses of food remnants and too many microorganisms, the objects of dental hygiene.

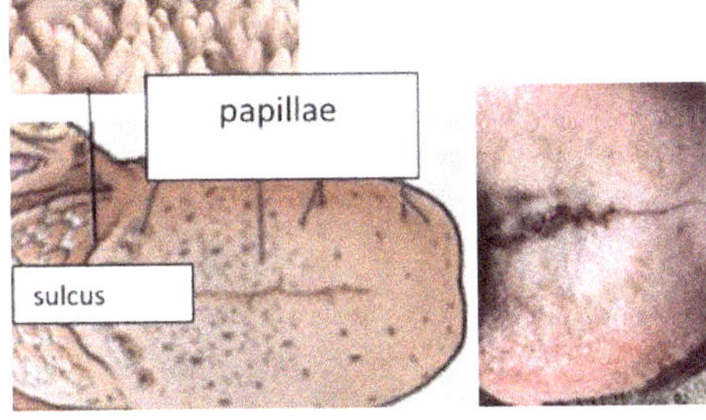

Median sulcus groove

The root contains predominantly tactile receptors in the middle, but at the sides are predominantly taste receptors, so-called fungiform papillae. These small, multiple papillae require gentle care. This difference is mentioned regarding pressure on the tongue during brushing.

The back of the tongue ends up almost vertically. It includes relatively large (7-12 mm) Vallate papillae. Taste buds are embedded in the papillae. After this area, the tongue goes down almost vertically, merging with the pharynx.

The taste buds of this area are applying the vomiting reflex, the last defense line protecting the gut from unsafe food intake. The vomiting reflex is on guard how far the toothbrush can go toward the nasopharynx area of the throat during tongue cleaning.

Besides vocalization and other functions, many short but vigorous tongue muscles actively control mouth content. These muscles' movements first reveal some interdental food remnants or just on gums. In this regard, as far as dental hygiene is concerned, maintaining the integrity of the tactile receptors while brushing the tongue should be kept in mind.

Physiology

The physiology of the teeth is apparently part of the physiology of the mouth, which, for the sake of simplification, can be limited to two main components: saliva and microbiome. Both components are major players in dental hygiene.

Saliva

Saliva's function is the starting point of the body's food-digesting chemical plant. Besides food lubrication and softening for more successful chewing, saliva serves only for following digestion preparation because there is not enough time for a finished product due to fast swallowing. However, the secretion of big pairs from both sides of glands (parotic, submandibular, sublingual) includes, among other enzymes, the alfa-amylase, which is designated for carbohydrate digestion metabolism. This circumstance should be taken into account while considering dental hygiene practices.

A healthy oral cavity generates a saliva flow of 0.4–0.5 ml/minute. Approximately 750 ml of saliva is secreted daily. Saliva works as a film that covers the oral cavity. Regarding oral hygiene, saliva functions such as the dilution of sugars after food intake, and the metabolism of remnants can be significant.

The commonly accepted theory is that stimulating saliva flow increases the acids washing out, as well as the concentration of bicarbonate buffer and demineralizing ions. When the saliva pH is below 5.5, tooth enamel can begin to dissolve. When the pH is above this value, saliva's calcium and phosphate ions start to repair any damaged mineral crystals in the enamel—the remineralization process. In healthy teeth, the loss of minerals is balanced by the reparative mechanisms of saliva.

The pH of dental plaque (biofilm) is a critical factor in the balance between acid demineralization of the teeth and the remineralization of the initial caries lesion if any occurs. Plaque pH falls each time acid accumulates due to bacterial acid production following consuming fermentable carbohydrates in foods. Plaque pH rises when the acids are washed away or neutralized by saliva containing the important buffer, bicarbonate.

Again, this is a commonly accepted theory. I doubt that the plague pH is measured with a reliable method. I also haven't seen experimental data on the saliva remineralization process.

Saliva is teeth protector, the first line of defense. However, under certain circumstances, which will be discussed in the following section, saliva's enzymatic activity can damage teeth health.

Microbiota

In contrast to anatomical data, where I have firsthand knowledge as an anatomical pathologist, and even some physiology awareness because saliva's alfa-amylase was part of my research study in the Ph.D. program, my knowledge is limited to reading appropriate dental microbiology literature, which I have to accept at face value.

Although they linger, I should suppress my doubts about the reliability of these data. I could not read the details of the methodology used to generate them.

Additional doubts about the reliability of dental science research data might be added to an email I received while writing this book on 7/19/23. The excerpt of this canned letter: *Dear Dr. Izak B. Dimenstein, Greetings from the "Journal of Dental and Oral Care". We appreciate your professionalism, deep insight, and understanding of the subject of dental and oral care after reading your article "The Concept of a Compound Autopsy Experimental Laboratory for SARS-CoV-2 Aerosolization Studies". We would like to invite you to submit your expert commentary/review articles based on your previous scientific endeavors..."*

Everyone can see how far my article's subject is from the journal's scope. The peer-review requirement might be softened due to the journal's hunger for submissions.

General notions

Let's go to the terms extracted from the literature and modern views. This theoretical background is essential. The description is tedious and, at first sight, redundant; however, I need it because otherwise, I cannot defend the personal dental hygiene principles, which, in my view, are rational, especially my insistence on details of actions.

Microbiota is now replacing the previous term for microflora. Microflora is an ancient term now used to differentiate a sub-group from the whole microbiota. Microflora is technically incorrect as the extrapolation of plant microorganisms for animal microorganisms. The microflora term, as more impressive, is better for visualization of the processes on the teeth and their mouth neighborhood. It can be used with microbiota terms interchangeably. The term 'germs' is preferably used for potential pathogens, while microflora is non-related to health issues.

The mouth is the first encounter place of the individual's alimentary canal with the outside world. Like the other microbiotas of the body (gut, skin, and vaginal), oral microbiota is a collection of microorganism groups that include bacteria, archaea, fungi, and viruses. The oral microbiota possesses them at the tongue, the hard palate, the teeth, the area around the tooth surfaces, and above and below the gums.

The oral cavity has many surfaces, and every surface encompasses a broad, diverse microbiota/microflora. Samples revealed more than 600 bacterial species.

Some microorganisms that colonize humans are commensal, meaning they co-exist without harming or benefiting humans. Certain microorganisms perform tasks that are known to be helpful. Conversely, some non-pathogenic microorganisms can harm human hosts via the metabolites that they produce. Only a small proportion of microorganisms are associated with disease or pathogenicity. The overwhelming majority of microbes are essential for healthy ecosystem functioning. The mouth microorganisms are their entire universe that live on complicated biological rules and features. Oral biologists discovered even gluten-degrading enzymes in microbes that live in the mouth.

This is just an example from a different microorganism's world. Wine microbiota includes wild flora (yeasts and bacteria), cultivated flora (yeasts), contamination flora (bad for taste, but none is pathogenic), and pathogens (mostly molds).

Oral microbiota/microflora attempts to colonize every possible location inside the oral cavity. Colonization leads to a microbial meshwork with specific members assigned to different locations.

Biofilm "anatomy"

The concept that microorganisms exist as single cells began to change as it became increasingly obvious that microbiotas occur within complex assemblages with species interaction.

Prokaryotes [cells without a nucleus] dwell in communities with several interacting species. The aggregating microbes are forming biofilms. The slimy coating on unbrushed teeth is a biofilm. Biofilms form when groups of bacteria cover themselves in a sticky mixture of sugars, proteins, and DNA. This extracellular matrix reversibly attaches by gluing bacteria to the tooth's surface and protects cells in the interior from outside "intruders." As the biofilm matures, bacteria specialize to perform different tasks within the biofilm.

According to the concept of *quorum sensing* (Bonnie Bassler's serial of studies, *Mol. Microbiol.* 1993; 9:773–786), cell-cell communication allows bacteria to control cooperative activities and adapt their phenotypes to the biotic environment, resulting in cell-cell adhesion or biofilm formation. Biofilm keeps related kin-selected individual bacteria close to each other. The bottom line is that bacterial biofilms, or plagues, the subject of prophylactic teeth and gum care, are complicated structures that have developed over millions of years of evolution. Biofilms existed before teeth arrived.

"Microbial condominium"

The College American Pathologists *CAPTODAY* publication (August 2023) quoted Dr. Versalovic, pathology professor, "It's [microbiota] about communities of cells, similar to any organ in the human's body."

 I would suggest the bacteria biofilms as an analogy of condominiums on a particular terrain (tooth) in an urban settlement, such as a city or township (mouth). They have their "bio bylaws" (my term). In contrast to the human condo's bylaws of the civilized world, the "bio bylaws" are more discriminatory. According to these "bio bylaws," kin selection surrounds each single bacteria with a similar genetic code, just as human condos are governed by a board of directors, which applies a high assessment fee in a gated high-cost private property. A settlement by a social outsider in such a community would be questionable, as the intrusion in biofilms dwelling at the teeth and mouth surfaces by dental hygiene hyperactivity can be counterproductive.

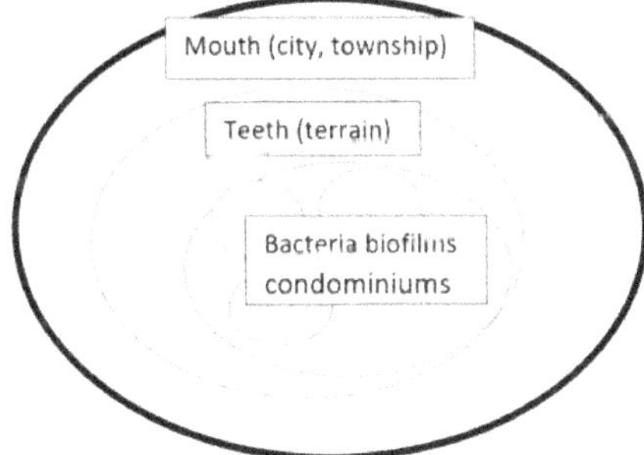

"Microbial condominium" diagram

Bacteria metabolism

Bacteria need organic molecules for carbon and energy. The energy-yielding catalytic reactions can be of different types. Sugar metabolism produces energy for the cell via two different processes: fermentation and respiration. The latter is more effective because fermentation is an anaerobic process without any external electron acceptor.

An organic compound, such as sugar or amino acid, is broken down into smaller organic molecules. During catabolic reactions, glucose is broken down into lactic, succinic, acetic, and formic acids, ethyl alcohol, carbon dioxide, and hydrogen gas, but the main one is lactic acid.

Is microbiota/microflora a friend or enemy for teeth, our jewel? Neither. Bacteria biofilms are just teeth' neighbors, part of other dwellers in the mouth, but the main part of them. A good neighbor sometimes helps to avoid some intruder pathogens. The excess of "ingredients" for bacterial metabolism provides a nutritional feast for benign or even pathological germs. When the neighborhood becomes overcrowded without relocation options, fences must be built, but it is better to do this in advance. This is the meaning of prophylactic teeth care and dental hygiene.

The significance to keep the evolutionary developed microbiota integrity can be shown on an example far from mouth. The bowel is prepared for a colonoscopy with a cleanser. It takes around two weeks to recover the colonic microbiota, essentially necessary for gut metabolism.

.

Special Part

Dental hygiene includes personal teeth and gum maintenance. It is related to but different from the professional service provided by dental hygienists in dental offices. Among the functions delegated by the dentist, the dental hygienist, hopefully, controls the quality of personal dental care and manages cleaning areas that a person cannot reach, such as the subgingival space.

This healthcare specialty has its principles of work and a set of special instruments. I've read the voluminous *Mosby's Comprehensive Review of Dental Hygiene* with interest while writing the current book. The manual calls a person with whom the dental hygienist works a client instead of a patient. This is right, in principle. Personal dental hygiene aims to reduce the number of patients in dental offices, which is one of the current book's aims.

Prophylactic tooth care is a commonly accepted part of oral hygiene and is described in many publications, including those written for the general public. However, while considering the general picture of teeth care, it would be reasonable to focus on the components with a clear understanding that it is an artificial divide.

This is the reason that only three areas of personal teeth care are discussed in this book's Special Part:

Enamel protection,

Caries prevention,

and Periodontal health.

Other individually essential subjects, for example, cosmetics or alveolar bone state considerations, are outside the topic of discussion in this book, although they will be mentioned just as parenthetical remarks in the appropriate place.

Without any doubt, the complicated mouth physiology remains in place during these prophylactic actions. It would not be a great revelation to say that people's cultural, dietary, and behavioral patterns affect their levels of individual tooth care in a specific area of their dwelling.

Enamel protection

Latin: *Enamelum;* Latin synonym: *Substantia adamantine*. An allusion is in the English phrase: "An adamant is an imaginary stone of impenetrable hardness."

The "theoretical" part of the enamel protection section is relatively large in this narrative to improve the reader's understanding of the background regarding the enamel's firmness and conditions of its damage. This description might support my take on the enamel protection issue from my experience as a pathology practitioner who has handled teeth regularly.

A little on enamel extracted from literature. It is necessary for a more meaningful explanation of my considerations. One of the main sources is *Lacruz RS, et al. Dental Enamel Formation and Implications for Oral Health and Disease. Physiol Rev* 97: 939 –993, 2017. Published by the American Physiological Society, the 55-page review includes 645 references. I read only some of them. The entire text was a pleasure to read as an example of scientific research. It required rereading to digest the scientific data.

Enamel as the "tooth skin"

Organs of the body that encounter the outside world use different kinds of protective epithelial shields (from Greek epi "upon"). Skin is an apparent visible example.

A tooth uses enamel, the mineralized epithelial cover, as an organ. Under normal conditions, enamel is the single example of mineralized epithelium in the body. Enamel covers the dentine cap of the crown of a tooth and serves as the wear-resistant outer layer.

As an epithelial structure, enamel follows the stratification principle of its elements' disposition. See cellular stratification enamel diagrams comparing with skin epithelium photo.

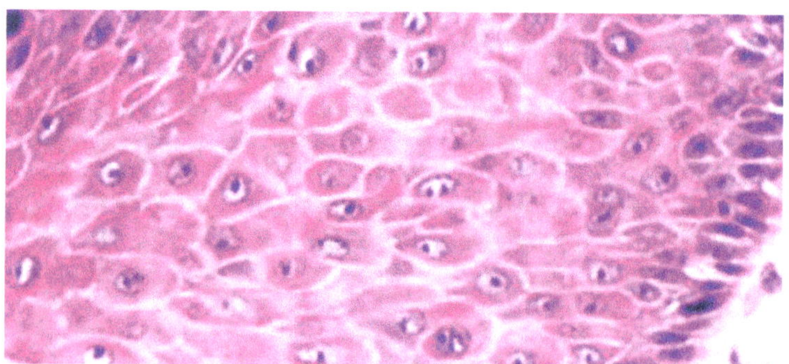

Skin epithelium

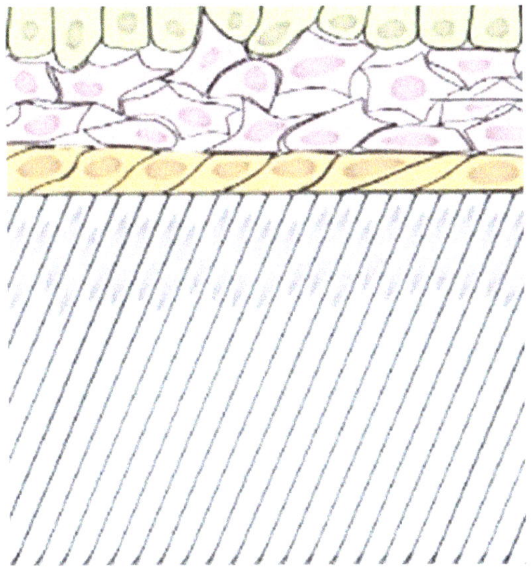

Enamel ameloblasts stratification. (Adapted from *Physiol Rev* 97: 939 –993, 2017.)

The thickness of enamel can be measured from specially prepared histological sections of teeth or high-resolution CT scans of teeth. Enamel layer thickness varies according to the type of tooth and anatomical location. It increases through the molar row towards the back of the mouth in all Hominids. The thickness of the enamel on the distal aspect was more significant than on the mesial aspect (the side of the tooth that's closest to the center of the mouth's arch) by an average of 0.10 mm. (I doubt the methodological base of this data, especially in the histological part).

Anyway, the enamel is a very thin layer, although on the diagrams it is presented as disproportionally thick. From the evolutionary point, the changes in the thickness of the enamel could not follow the speed in dietary opportunities after natural selection in human evolution has been stopped and replaced by artificial selection through adaptation to specific conditions of the dwelling.

According to the Mohs Scale of Hardness, tooth Dental enamel scores 5-6 (For reference, Diamond 10, Porcelain 6-7, Apatite 5, Gypsum 2). This means that it is almost as hard or harder than steel. Diamonds are the strongest substance on Earth. Being harder than steel, the enamel breaks much more easily. Enamel has little effect on tooth color, largely determined by dentine's properties.

Teeth enamel should not be confused with enamel in jewelry art products or both. Enameling is a process by which powdered glass is fused to a metal substrate at high heat.

 The Russian Rostov Veliky finift enamel

Enamel provides maximum durability that allows teeth to function as weapons (rarely by humans now) and/or tools (crazy by some humans now) as well as for food processing (in the mouth kitchen). It forms an insulating barrier that protects the tooth's underlying dental pulp from mechanical, thermal, and chemical forces.

Enamel formation

This part is adapted to some extent from the review mentioned above. Although it is based on animal studies, many positions can be extrapolated to humans with prophylactic care applications while considering significant anatomy, physiology, and diet differences. However, the physiological process and general chemistry are the same. A reader can omit this part, but I need it to support my suggestion for prophylactic care applications.

The process of enamel formation is referred to as amelogenesis. Ameloblasts secrete enamel matrix proteins. These heavily polarized cells form a monolayer around the developing enamel tissue. They move into the enamel space as a single forming front in specified directions. They lay down a proteinaceous matrix that serves as a template for crystal growth while later degraded and proteolytically removed by ameloblasts. Ameloblasts maintain intercellular connections, creating a semi-permeable barrier that receives nutrients and ions from blood vessels at one end (basal/proximal) and, at the opposite end (secretory/apical/distal), forms extracellular crystals. Ameloblasts set up crystal growth via multiple cellular activities, including the transport of minerals and ions within specified pH conditions.

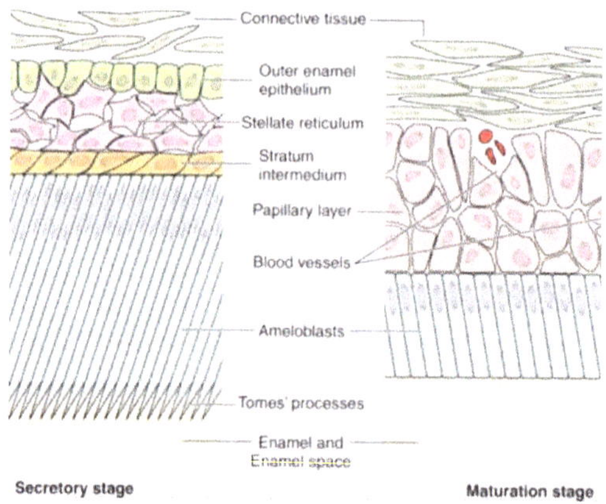

Adapted from Physiology Review 97: 939 –993, 2017
American Physiological Society.

Minute crystallites that are organized into bundles of approximately 6 micrometers in diameter prisms/rods. Crystallite orientation changes within prisms in a way determined by the shape of the cell processes of the secretory ameloblasts - the so-called Tomes process. This portion of the cytoplasm is filled with secretory granules containing the substance of the enamel matrix. After the ameloblasts complete the enamel deposition, they enter the maturation stage. The formed enamel has a prismatic appearance composed of rods, each formed by a single ameloblast and extending from the dentine-enamel junction (DEJ) to the enamel surface. The interrod enamel is located around the enamel rods. The cells then secrete more minerals on the enamel while absorbing most proteins. By weight, mature enamel is ~95% mineral, ~1–2% organic material, and ~2– 4% water.

Enamel mineralization

Tooth enamel is mostly hydroxyapatite, which is a mineral form of calcium phosphate. Ameloblasts regulate the formation of hydroxyapatite-based inorganic material within the enamel space. Apatite formation occurs under the formula:

$$10Ca^{2+} + 6HPO4^{2-} + 2H_2O \rightarrow Ca_{10}(PO_4)\,6(OH)_2 + \mathbf{8H^+}$$

The release of **$8H^+$** (hydrogen protons) is important because it means that the process requires the involvement of neutralizing factors to keep the reaction under neutral conditions of 6-7 pH. The 8H+ in bold anions is emphasized because they are participants in the demineralization process, which is discussed later.

According to the review mentioned above, the process is complicated and involves the use of active bicarbonate-(HCO^{3-} transport systems to regulate the extracellular pH, which is not of interest to our subject of enamel protection because we are dealing with the final product, namely apatite, enamel crystal. Our concern is opposite to the ameloblast cells' mineralization problems.

Under physiological conditions, apatite has the lowest solubility among the calcium phosphate minerals. It is the most chemically stable mineral in the human body's mineralized tissues. Hydroxyapatite ($Ca_{10}(PO_4)\,_6(OH)_2$) commonly has hexagonal symmetry in its crystal lattice.

However, there are calcium-deficient carbonated apatite and calcium-deficient carbonated hydroxyapatite. The first releases 4H+ and the second $12H^+$ protons. It means a different resistance acid environment, which is our enamel protection subject. Carbonated apatite is much more susceptible to acidic dissolution and dissolves at around 5 pH. Moreover, the exchange of CO_4^{3-} for F^- in fluorohydroxyapatite lowers the solubility.

Enamel prophylactic care

As seen on previous pages, enamel apatite formation is complex, and one should not rush with superficial recommendations. Moreover, due to numerous developmental variations, one should refrain from extrapolating some experiences as a norm or jumping to conclusions based on a singular experience.

Unlike bone, enamel tissue, once mineralized, is acellular. Enamel cannot regenerate itself. In this regard, the mechanism of enamel remineralization after demineralization described in the literature is difficult to comprehend.

Enamel damage can be twofold: mechanical forces breaking the continuity of thin layers and chemical "corrosion" of the apatite crystal lattice. Both processes are bounded. Regarding enamel protection issues, the mechanical event is primary, while in caries cases, the chemical process is the main.

Breaks of continuity

The mature enamel has unique morphological and biomechanical properties. In contrast with skin, which as the outer epithelial cover serves for protection from different kinds of environmental conditions, the enamel is designed to withstand mechanical challenges.

The skin has simple vertical stratification with loose intracellular connections. It can shed its epithelial cells under physiological conditions with the following replacement: Enamel is destined to keep its sophisticated design of calcified rods, which have some degree of flexibility to adjust the pressure of mechanical power during the chewing of hard substances, with the final response delegated to the periodontal ligament.

When both fail, a problem might occur under certain conditions of teeth alignment in the jaws' alveolar bone. Enamel also has a crack deflection toughening mechanism at the orientation of the nanoscale crystals, which can fail.

Unlike stainless steel in enamel jewelry, tooth enamel is not monolithic and is prone to chipping away in some spaces due to mechanical pressure. Visible or, in most cases, invisible cracks in the continuity of the enamel's surface are the failure of the first line of defense. It is common knowledge that tooth enamel is brittle.

Initial damage on the enamel surface is often observed as "white spots" which illustrate that the organized mineral layer in enamel has been altered by a demineralization/remineralization process that most likely has been triggered by cariogenic acids produced by bacteria in the oral environment. White spot lesions or incipient caries consist of a demineralized zone covered by a superficial mineral layer often comprised of larger apatite crystals, which reflect light and, therefore, appear white. The common treatment for those lesions is fluoride, often as an acidulated gel or dentifrice.

A practical suggestion is not to challenge this line for casual habit, fan, or occasion, even by not popping out popcorn kernels. Do not try to open a beer bottle with your teeth, although some do. It's just my guess, but grainy bread with hardly chewable seeds might not be completely innocent of causing enamel micro-cracks in individuals predisposed to weak enamel.

I do not aim to touch the professional dentistry realm, but every revealed during professional exam white spot or other signs of minimal breaks in enamel continuity should be taken by a person seriously because it is the way for demineralization, which is the main subject for the following pages.

Demineralization

Enamel demineralization prevention is an apparent goal of prophylactic teeth care. All previous pages about enamel formation should give the readers of this brochure some clues about how tedious was the work of ameloblasts to prevent demineralization of this wonder of nature.

In the *Decalcification* chapter of my book *Grossing Bones: Principles, Techniques, Instruments* (Amazon.com, 2017), I explained this process in detail. Here's a diagram from the book.

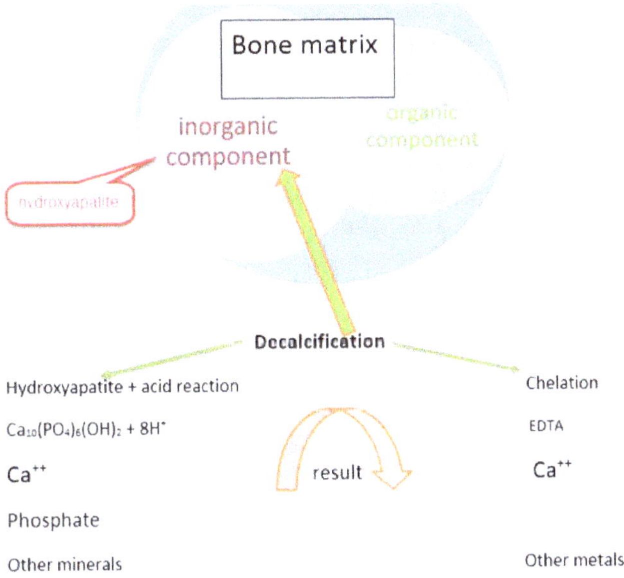

I always failed to make a dissent gross section of a tooth because enamel resisted demineralization while using formic acid on the rest of the tooth, a relatively weak acid. Enamel requires a strong acid, like hydrochloric. The **8H+** protons released during apatite formation must react in the opposite direction.

Sometimes, even scientific publications mention the chelation process in tooth demineralization. It has nothing to do with real physiological conditions in the mouth. EDTA (Ethylenediaminetetraacetic Acid) works as a chelating factor under neutral or higher than 8 pH, which is impossible on the teeth' surface.

I'm not going to go further on other details.

While considering many possible precipitating factors, such as genetic predisposition, defects in enamel formation, fluctuating fluoride exposition, and others, two main well-known culprits can be suspected: diet and microbiota/microflora (the bacteria part of it).

The trick is that they work in concert. The broken enamel precipitates their nefarious behavior in the mouth as the first line of defense. Discussing them in the next section about caries makes sense, especially because, as I already mentioned, separating these chapters was artificial to concentrate on the particularities of enamel's protection details.

Remineralization occurs when essential minerals like fluoride, calcium, and phosphate reunite in a person's enamel. The demineralization and remineralization processes are likely going in parallel under physiological conditions. However, in my view, it would be wrong to imitate the natural biological process with pastes, rinses, or other "patches" on the teeth enamel "wounds" of demineralization artificially unless we have credible experimental data of positive outcomes of such efforts. I'm discussing only the prevention of further demineralization.

In conclusion, given my personal experience handling teeth and their enamel covering, I find it difficult to believe that weak acids in the mouth can demineralize the enamel to a clinically significant degree unless a precondition exists, like a tiny, even invisible crack or disturbances in an organism's mineral biochemistry, among other reasons. These unknown circumstances justify an individual's dental hygiene routine.

Do not challenge the toughness of your tooth enamel

Soft drinks and enamel demineralization

I want to discuss one issue related to enamel deterioration, which is blamed on carbonized drinks because it is popular and controversial. Although soft drinks are accused of caries, the enamel is definitely the first line of defense.

I want to touch on this subject from different aspects.

Chemical aspect

Soda, or fizzy drinks, is carbonated water with numerous additions depending on the brand. Water and carbon dioxide (CO_2) are placed in a tightly sealed container. During carbonization, carbon dioxide gas is injected into the water at a pressure of 1200 pounds per inch for commercial distribution. This process can be imitated at home from a loaded CO_2 charger canister. The gas was placed into a canister under pressure.

Upon reaching water, carbon dioxide gas becomes carbon acid H_2CO_3. It remains in this acid aggregate state until it is released when the container is opened in form of Carbone dioxide (fuzzy babbles) and water. Diagram illustrates the chemical process.

$$H_2CO_3 \rightleftarrows CO_2 + H_2O \quad \text{chemical reaction}$$

Carbonized drinks

$$CO_2 + H_2O \text{ under pressure} \Longrightarrow H_2CO_3 \text{ release} \Longrightarrow CO_2 + H_2O$$

soft drink in can/bottle   bubbles in wet mouth

Yes, soda cans and bottles contain dissolved carbonic acid (H_2CO_3). Researchers measured pH in acidic brackets around 3-4. But for the enamel demineralization justification, it is an exercise in futility because people have not the acid but carbon gas (CO2) and water (H2O) in their mouths, which are swallowed and go out during breath while mixing with the exhaled carbon dioxide. There is no time for a chemical reaction.

More chemistry is significant for evaluating soft drinks' acidity regarding enamel demineralization.

The acidity of a soft drink cannot be represented only by pH. pKa (acid dissociation constant) reflects dissolution, which is how the acid dissolves into its ions. Carbonic acid is in the weak acids category. It is stronger (by pH and pKa) than the physiologically important lactic acid and almost three times weaker than pyruvic acids. Both are the end products of carbohydrate bacterial metabolism. In contrast with carbonic acid, these acids stay in the mouth.

A remarkable example. Hydrofluoric acid (HF) is very corrosive and used for etching; it is a weak acid. It is not free to function as an acid in water (pKa 3.18), while pKa of strong acids like sulfuric acid -10 or hydrochloric acid -7.

Physical aspect

Just common sense. Nobody gurgles a soft drink. Food/drink enters the gut. The acid in a soft drink's gas (CO_2) is breathed out.

Physiology aspect

Immediately upon taking the fuzzy drink, the mouth's taste receptors signal the salivary glands that something admirable has arrived. The glands react enthusiastically by producing neutral buffering saliva to bring the pH close to neutral.

Studies reliability

Unfortunately, I haven't encountered any satisfactory scientific study on this subject from the methodological aspect. An example of a recently published review in *Nutrients*. 2023 Apr 6;15(7): 1785. *Damage from Carbonated Soft Drinks on Enamel*. 100 references were included in this study. They were completely different from the initial data collection methodology.

The review came to the following conclusion, which is cited entirely: *"A Systematic Review Boolean a binary variable, having two possible values called "true" and "false." An abuse of carbonated acid substances leads to an increase in the possibility of dental erosion with consequent structural disintegration and reduction of the physical and mechanical properties of the enamel. The pH of most commercialized carbonated drinks is lower than the critical pH for the demineralization of the enamel. Carbonated drinks' pH and duration of exposure have different deleterious effects on enamel duration of the demineralization process."*

Completely inconclusive result of the study.

Juices, especially with pulp, are more significant in the acidic mouth environment than sodas, but not for demineralizing enamel. I believe additional unfavorable conditions should be considered for the damaging effect of citric juices. For example, some people should take into account already-existing caries because the acidic content is trapped there.

From my experience demineralizing bones in the histology laboratory described above, I understood that this is a prolonged process, especially with weak acids, completely opposite to soft drink consumption. At the end of my workshops on bone demineralization, I sometimes asked the audience: Can Coca-Cola dissolve iron? Only a few people responded confidently, "No." Urban legends linger.

Caries prevention

Dental caries is a biofilm-mediated, diet-modulated, multifactorial, non-communicable, dynamic disease resulting in net mineral loss of dental hard tissues. This is the consensus workshop definition of caries published in the *Caries Research journal (2020, 54 (1): 7–14).*

In contrast with enamel, which sounds like a woman's name and is certainly part of women's jewelry, caries has always had a negative connotation. A decay of a seemingly firm structure like a bone. A hole, in general parlance. This was correct because caries was revealed before the x-ray was implemented in every dental office, usually in the late stage. A cavity, actually a cave, where something nefarious occurs.

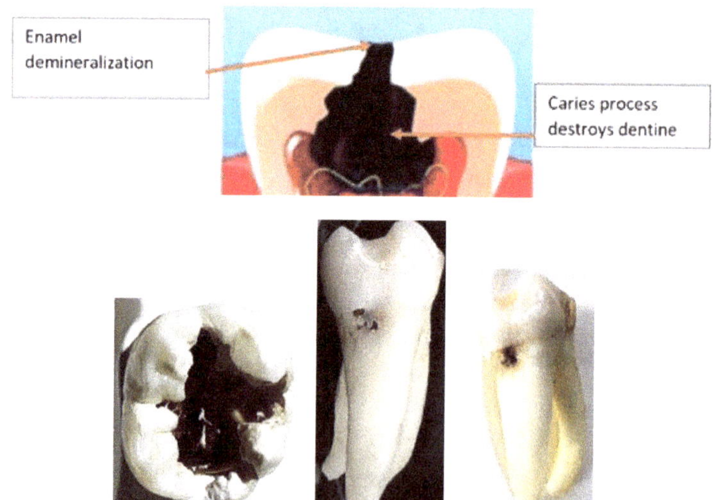

Introductory remarks

In this book, I will not attempt a review on caries, which is the realm of dentistry's cariology discipline. Many professional organizations are for this purpose. There is the American Academy of Cariology. The Cariology Research Group (CRG) is one of the numerous scientific groups of the International Association for Dental Research (IADR) and perhaps others.

Moreover, while I could even touch enamel during my professional work, tooth caries is a subject on which I have to rely on the experience of practitioners, scientific data, and the hope that the interpretation of the data does not involve too much imagination.

As in the enamel case, I haven't encountered a study with regular histology serial sections of caries lesions. I've seen only macro photos, radiology, and diagrams. I have an explanation for this absence, but it would be out of the scope of this book.

Caries development

Dental science and practice have concluded that tooth caries' culprits are acids and proteolytic enzymes, the final products of bacteria carbohydrate metabolism. These enzymes do demineralization work on a tooth's *apatite* mineral content.

Streptococcus mutans was named the main intruder many years ago. Streptococcus sobrinus and Lactobacilli were also isolated from advanced caries. The ecological plaque hypothesis suggests that a specific type of microorganism does not cause dental caries but results from a shift in the microbiota of the dental biofilm towards more cariogenic species. Oral biofilm from healthy teeth has a higher diversity than from carious teeth.

The inciting event is the deposition of bacteria plaque (biofilm) on the tooth. Of course, it is more complicated. There are also different paradigms of the process, for example, the role of fluoride in the pathogenesis of the disease. Yes, it is a disease, though often without prominent manifestation.

Without going further into the murky forest of the pathogenesis or theoretical background of caries, I would like to present some of the literature's understanding of individual prophylactic attempts to prevent or diminish caries development in this book. Such attempts resemble enamel protection in general, to some degree depending on the latter, but they require more specifics in food consumption and actions.

Prophylactic principles

The principle of caries prophylactic is in the rationing of the leftovers allocated for the metabolism of even friendly bacteria, for their ability to build a protective biofilm for the teeth and gums. The rationing should be limited to minimize the situation that the byproduct of their fermentation process, namely acids (lactic acid especially), would start demineralization of enamel and dentin under certain unfortunate conditions (crack, fluoride deficiency or overdose, etc. too many).A person finishes food consumption with more or less a taste feast. Still, the mouth-inhabitant bacteria and other members of the microflora are waiting hungrily for their part. And here starts the conflict of interests.

In general, the type of food does not matter in the initial stage of consumption in the mouth, where food preparation occurs for the gut. Chewing and preparing the bolus for swallowing takes so little time that bacteria and other mouth inhabitants can't arrange any nefarious reaction. They rely on leftovers. Individual food consumption depends on many factors that cannot and should not be directly related to caries prevention. Habits, diet, taste, chewing abilities, and many other details are in play. However, prophylactic measures should be taken depending on the type of food used in concrete food consumption situations. It would sound like a travesty that starch-rich bread, predominately protein in meat, and only fiber pieces of lettuce require a different treatment after they leave the mouth.

I want to add personal bias to the kind of food regarding caries prevention considerations. This stems from my experience of amylase enzyme testing during my work in science in the PhD program. Now I remember how fast the starch became hydrolyzed when the tested blood or urine sample was added under body-temperature incubation (the iodometric Amyloclastic method). Related to the caries prevention issue, this circumstance might play a role under conditions of already-developed predisposition to caries.

Saliva can start to supply bacteria with highly desired carbohydrate fragments. Under demineralization conditions when Ca++ ions are in play, the alfa-amylase activity increases.

After presenting these general positions, I would formulate my two basic suggestions:

The teeth area should be cleaned from food by means available in the concrete life situation.

The mouth should be empty from any food between meals as much as possible by the lifestyle.

Caries prevention is not the goal of life. It cannot be a kind of obsession, but washing hands before a meal is a habit of civilization. In the same way, at least rinsing the mouth after a meal, if the conditions allow, would be another right habit. In particular, civilized life provides appropriate conditions.

Clear your mouth from remnants of food

Periodontium health

This section will be short for many reasons. There is little to suggest more besides what has been said in two previous sections regarding prophylactic dental care. Individual prophylactic actions differ from the professional hygienist's prophylaxis and have nothing to do with professional periodontal maintenance. If suggested in the ideal case, they should be the reinforcement extension of home care according to individual recommendations.

Nevertheless, I would like to present some remarks related to periodontium health issues. Maintaining periodontal health includes measures to prevent periodontitis because, apparently, treatment of it is the failure of prophylactic.

Reminder from the *Anatomy* section

Teeth sit in the jaw bone but do not directly touch the bone. They are embedded into the periodontal ligament (PDL). Like a part of suspension in a car, it is a continuation of enamel's function designed to withstand vertical and shear forces during chewing. The periodontal ligament opens to the outside world (the mouth) with a gingival sulcus, as a part of the gingiva, but very fragile, covered with a thin layer of non-keratinized squamous epithelium. This construction is vulnerable to trauma due to sulcus blood and tissue debris collection.

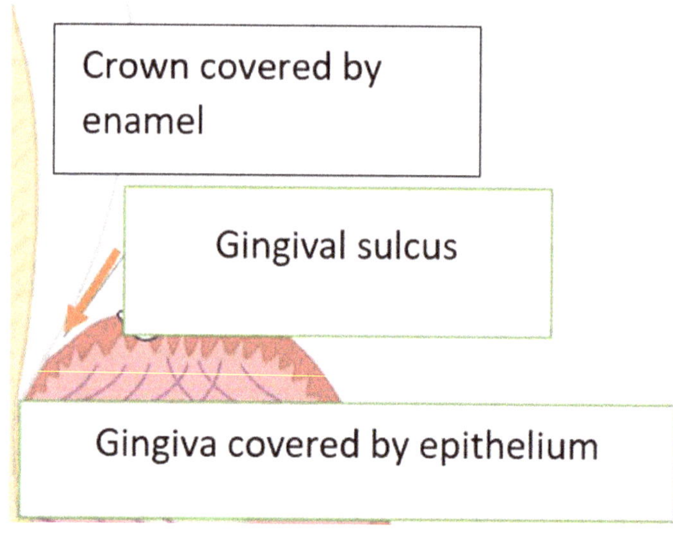

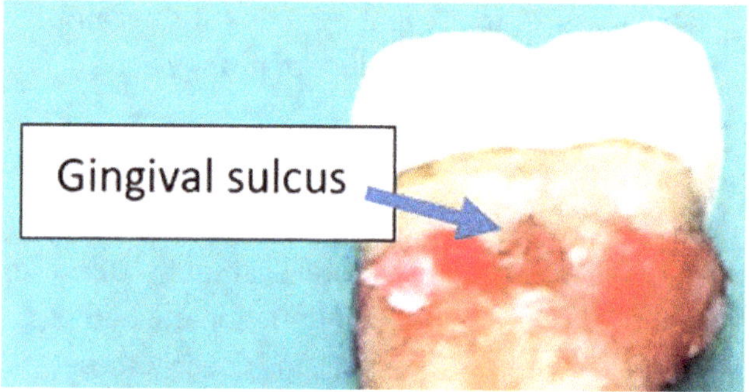

Remnant of gingival sulcus of an extracted tooth.

The gingival sulcus, 0.5-to 2 mm grove, is, in my view, the battleground of maintaining periodontal health. Otherwise, the sulcus would become a periodontal pocket, even with the loss of the periodontal ligament, which cannot be easily regenerated due to periodontal inflammation.

Preserving the integrity of the gingival sulcus and periodontal ligament is the key to periodontal health. From the preventive dental care perspective, mechanical, sharp devices for cleaning interdental space should not be used. Vegetables and other food stuck between teeth should be removed with gentle efforts.

Besides mechanical injuries, which ought to be avoided by any means, even vigorous brushing might damage the thin epithelial layer of the sulcus. By the way, the tongue is the first tool because it works in a proper direction, especially for lower jaw teeth.

Some details regarding periodontal ligament protection will be discussed later in the Methods and Tools part.

Bacteria, which are commonly understood and even found in dental offices, have a bad reputation in regard to dental health. They are considered hooligans or even terrorists. In the Microbiota section, I've tried presenting modern views on this subject. Bacteria and other microbiota/microflora inhabitants of teeth and gums are the product of millions of years of evolution.

However, change occurred when the industry made processed sugar and flour readily available. Oral microbial diversity plummeted, and the main caries-causing microbe, *Streptococcus mutans*, became dominant. We should take this into account when performing our prophylactic actions.

We don't disinfect our dishes, we clean them. Food left on the plate is for the microorganisms' festive.

Healthy teeth/mouth does not need disinfection. Intrusion is microorganism environment only way to periodontal disease than prevention of it. My point is Sanitation vs. Disinfection

 According to *the Mosby's Comprehensive Review of Dental Hygiene* textbook for hygienists, "*Successful of professional care depends on the control of bacterial plague; therefore, instruction and supervision in plague removal procedures for a daily participation by the client [individual] precedes, continues simultaneously with, and follows instrumentation by the clinician [hygienist].*"

 I placed this quote in its entirety to encourage the potential client/individual before being offered by the clinician/hygienist the ugly sharp instruments (scalers, curettes) to do homework. From this quote, I also took an understanding that everything comes eventually to fight bacterial plague.

Bacteria are friends but kept at bay

Parenthetical remark

Before moving to the Methods and Tools part, I want to make a parenthetical remark. While preparing the current book, I dove into the dental care literature and science that support the main postulates. I tried to find morphology data, especially histology data, closer to my knowledge.

Remarkably, scientists go from schemes and diagrams directly to electron microscopy illustrations, as in the abovementioned review on enamel, without presenting the same area in a histology section. I haven't seen a histology section of bone buildup around a dental implant; only diagrams are usually demonstrated. In my view, the problem with dentistry science histology is the technical difficulties of demineralization, while working with unmineralized teeth brings other issues.

A decent grossing sample and, eventually, a micro section require some tricks in processing. While in maxillofacial surgery, a tooth sits in the alveolar socket, a separate extracted tooth needs secure immobilization for a grossing section. In the book *Grossing Bones: Principles, Techniques, Instruments*, I discussed this problem and some ways to resolve it.

Without serious experimental morphological support, dentistry science will remain at the level of assumptions. Molecular biology methods also require reliable initial materials. The histology section is a basic starting point and proof of the area that molecular biology studies reflect

Methods and Tools

With definite simplification, all prophylactic individual teeth care methods can be divided into three main procedures:

teeth brushing

interdental cleaning/flossing

mouth rinsing.

All three main procedures will be discussed separately for the detailed presentation in the current book. This separation is artificial. Moreover, there could be numerous deviations from the presented methods in real life depending on individual preferences, time, and life circumstances.

In this book, I discuss prophylactic personal teeth care following the pattern of setting the goal of the procedure while explaining the reason for the procedure as much as I can.

What/Why. By presenting the optimal, in my view, method or methods for achieving the goal, I'll try to show

How to do it using the best

With, in my judgment, tools to give a systematic approach by following this pattern of the individual prophylactic teeth care presentation.

All prophylactic teeth/mouth care actions should have an **Out** direction with minimal **In** occasions. The different shapes of the circles in the diagram should clarify this premise

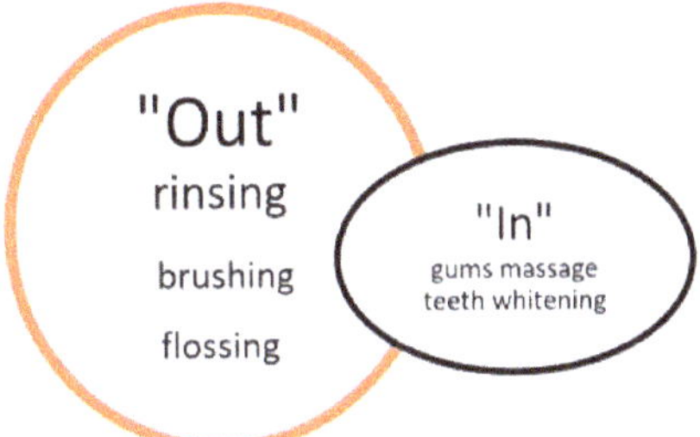

Appeal for details

I have some sense of humor regarding the distance of subjects by invoking Georgio Armani's famous phrase about the importance of details: To create something exceptional, your mindset must be relentlessly focused on the smallest detail. I'm using it to draw attention to the details of personal dental hygiene procedures. Moreover, it is well known that things people encounter as routine often go unnoticed. And the devil laughs while watching how those neglected details nullify noble intentions and endeavors.

This appeal to pay attention to the details stems from my bitter experience of numerous failures in clinical research and experimental immunology when neglected methodology details led to inconclusive results. Put differently, I have found from my practice in the surgical pathology histology laboratory that only scrupulous attention to detail provides consistent results.

Toothbrushing

Introductory words

Translating energetic vigorous English "brushing teeth" into more precise German's Zähneputzen somehow clarifies one of the main individual prophylactic teeth care procedures as simply teeth cleaning. However, a question remains: What is cleaning from? In contrast to washing your hands, I would have difficulty explaining to a curious child the action we try to implement as a routine habit. Brushing hair would be a much easier task to explain.

With sincere apology to these great professions, a brush, with all the ridiculousness of the comparison, is like a surgeon's, plumber's, or cook's tool for a procedure whose goal is not clearly defined. Cleaning of what? The teeth and mouth are degraded to a container, aviating a toothbrush as a waste truck.

The previous pages tried to show that teeth and mouth, evolutionary product constructions, live their own lives, and every intrusion in them requires understanding and respect. Individuals need these intrusions, including brushing, to prolong the durability of teeth and mouth construction and adjust to the modern dwelling style. I want to repeat and summarize my views on the goals of "cleaning." Repetition is not ignored in classical and modern music.

Toothbrushing as part of individual dental care

The American Academy of Pediatric Dentistry (AAPD) and the American Academy of Pediatrics (AAP) issued recommendations for at-home preventive measures within 6 months of the eruption of the first tooth and no later than 12 months old, including brushing infants and young children's teeth and using fluoride toothpaste.

The American Dental Association (ADA) and the British Dental Association (BDA) recommend brushing teeth twice daily for two minutes with a soft-bristled toothbrush and an ADA-accepted fluoride toothpaste.

Why twice a day?

When is appropriate tooth brushing during the day?

Why two minutes?

I could not find independent cohort randomized studies on these recommendations. Perhaps they exist, but I could not find them. Perhaps the dental organizations just approved the common practice.

What/why

Food comes and goes. The individual's body needs it, and the teeth/mouth microbiota population's metabolism needs it as a useful scavenger that does his sanitary work on leftovers.

The "cleaning" rationale is to keep microflora activities at bay by rationing ingredients for their metabolism, especially carbohydrates—more details in previous sections.

Brushing teeth in the morning aims to eliminate unpleasant taste/odor after the microbiota crowd in the mouth and make too many byproducts during their uninterrupted sleeping person metabolism activities.

Brushing in the evening is determined by leaving this crowd with less food and leftover ammunition for these activities. The two-minute duration of the procedure reflects the time that a person, on average, is willing to allocate for it.

A clear understanding of the brushing procedure's goal might determine many practical actions. Hopefully, the previous pages provided my "theoretical" background.

Twice a day is obligatory, and after every meal is desirable. It matters after any meal or is discriminatory, depending on the components. It does matter immediately after a meal, but it depends on life circumstances. By the way, there is a notion (British Dental Association) to wait at least 60 minutes.

How

Below are technical descriptions of the teeth brushing procedure. I'm using the word "procedure" intentionally to emphasize the importance of details.

General considerations

The principle of teeth brushing is to remove the object of "cleaning" from the teeth' surfaces, especially from anatomical pockets. Most people practice the just horizontal movement of the brush back and force along the teeth. But this is not optimal. Moreover, in some occasions, depending on the construction of teeth and their place in the alveolar ridge is counterproductive. This type of brushing certainly requires flossing because some tiny fragments inevitably get stuck between the teeth.

Initially

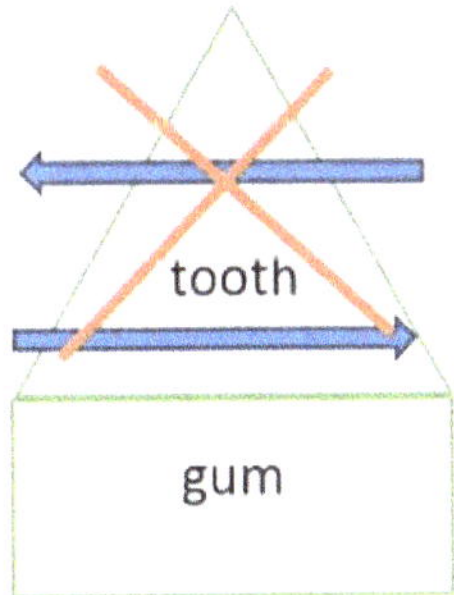

except whitening, this is a different procedure in its goals and methods.

The brush moves down from the gum on the upper jaw, but it moves up on the lower jaw.

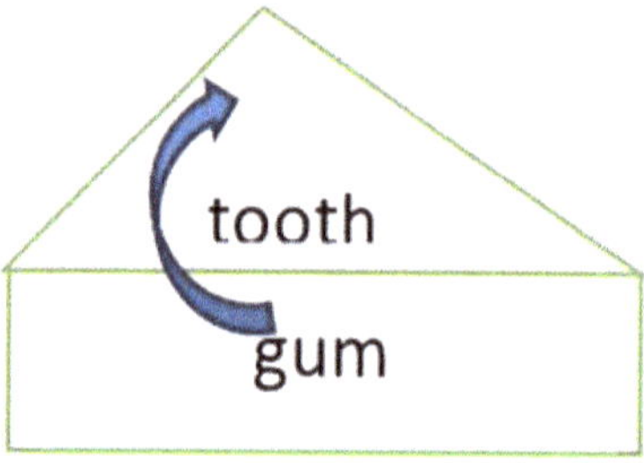

For the lower jaw.

According to the toothpaste fluoride application theory, fluoride can penetrate biofilm plague (bactericide ability) and other positive features. Some energetic horizontal movements would not hurt as a final action with teeth. Moreover, this would prolong the paste's presence in the mouth and generate more foam as a precondition for effective rinsing.

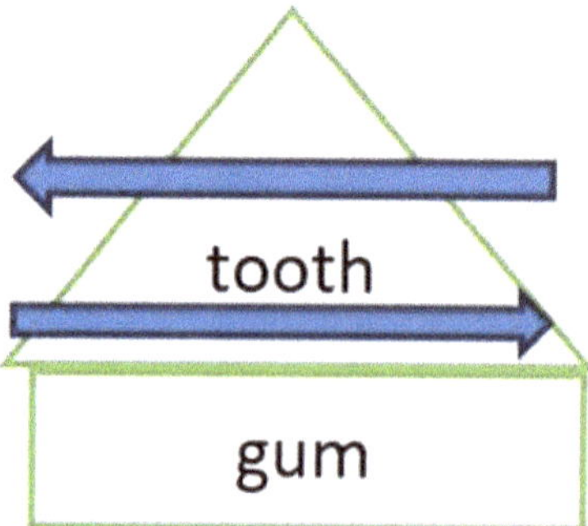

Two final movements before rinsing.

Brushing technique

With an apology for the travesty and repetitions of my descriptions. The wet, pasted-up toothbrush is held at a 45-degree angle to the gums, which means it is a little askew. The brush moves in short circular motions without much pressure, gentle at the gum line and more energetic to the end of the tooth. It is similar to sweeping a floor with a broom.

The time spent brushing also depends on tooth shape, skill, and temperament. The main point is establishing a pattern or sequence routine to ensure every tooth receives fair treatment.

Brushing sequence scheme

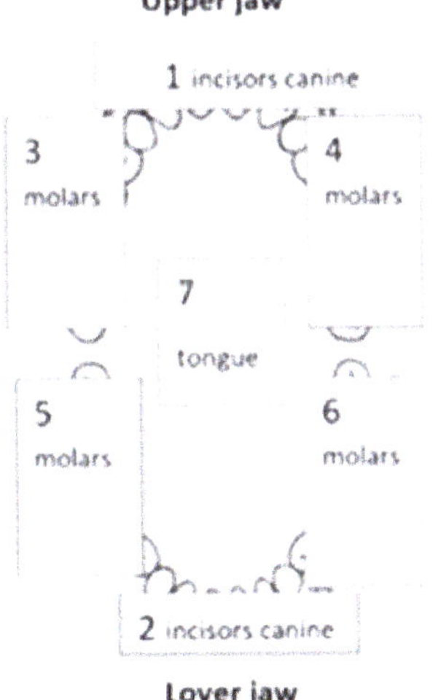

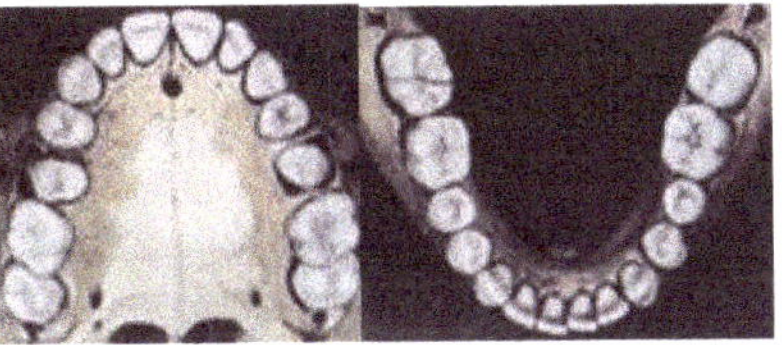

Upper jaw   Lower jaw

There could be differences in recommendations for the sequence of the tooth groups for brushing, using different parts of the brush for different groups. For example, the tip of the toothbrush head could be used to brush the lingual or back surfaces of the upper front teeth.

From right or left does not matter. What does matter is the standard in a person's head for automatic actions that assures all teeth involved in this ritualistic enterprise today, tomorrow, and after a year. Initial military training includes endless repetition of the same actions. Brushing teeth is the time to think about today's chores or something else while doing this procedure.

Start with the front teeth, incisors, and canines. They are less "contaminated" by food leftovers. Doing this from outside and inside surfaces would be easy by flicking a motion from the gum line toward the teeth's top.

Then, follow with the premolars and molars. Brushing from the gum line for the upper jaw teeth strokes down, arch brush movements go up in sweeping motions for the lower jaw. It is more difficult to hold the toothbrush parallel to the teeth line without missing every tooth. Brushing the premolars and molars should be finished with the top biting surfaces. This procedure is due to occlusion eminences, or cusps, which do the grinding work. The photo below reminds us of them.

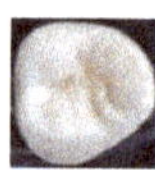 Molar's cusps.

As mentioned, the molar's hills and ravines at the surface are possible collections of food remnants, especially starch ingredients. By the way, the tip of the tongue (tactile receptors) is one of the first quality controls for clearing the cusps.

The molars' cusps are usually cleaned with circular brush movements because these grinding teeth are prone to storing food leftovers between cusps. Brushing molars requires more time due to the molar's surface, "hills terrane." It would be reasonable to rinse the brush and apply another thin paste layer after every right/left cleaning, but it is not obligatory.
It would also be right to periodically check your teeth with a mirror.

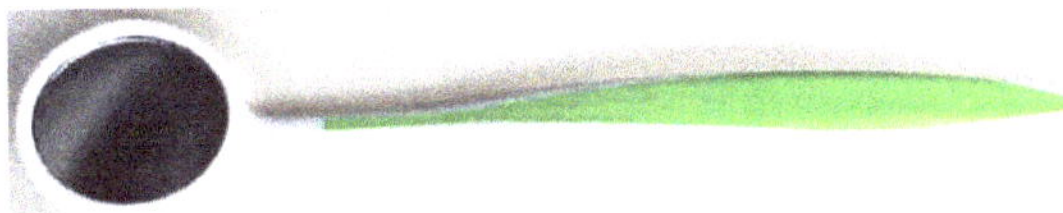

The toothbrushing procedure should be finished with tongue cleaning once a day.

With

Tools for teeth brushing are so numerous that I am afraid to be in the advertising swamp. I will mention only their design and use principles that seem to align with achieving the goals described above. There are two participants: toothbrushes and kinds of toothpaste. I'll express only my attitude towards them.

Toothbrushes

Since Du Pont Laboratories introduced nylon bristles toothbrushes in the 1930s, the design has remained the same with numerous shape variations, such as circular bristles, with rows of bristles in different heights and colors. There are multi-level bristles to reach different areas of the tooth surface. The bristles' materials range from castor-oil-based polymers and traditional petroleum-derived nylon polymers, Nylon and rubber, and Polybutylene terephthalate (PBT) fibers.

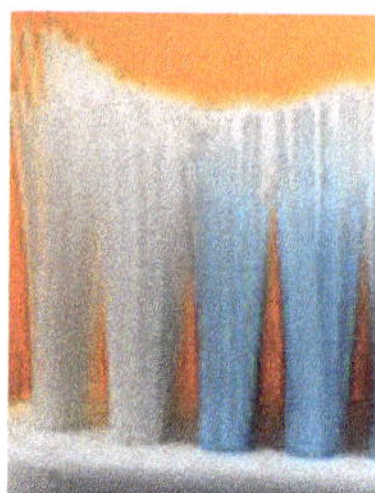 Standard toothbrush

By the way, I haven't seen a toothbrush with boar or badger bristles widely used for shavings or hair brushes. They would generate a rich lather that is important when using a paste.

The badger shavings brushes create a foamy content, perhaps due to emulsification by the lipofilling design of the badger's hair. More than likely, there are reasons that they are not used in toothbrushing. Again, in my view, brushing is preparation for intensive rinsing of foamy "dirty" content after manipulations with the teeth.

I prefer soft bristle toothbrushes. They are better than brushes with more rigid bristles in "cleaning" but presumably less traumatic. Micro bleeding of traumatized gums can be a source of collection of extra bacteria debris at the gingival sulcus area. Gums are not a dirty wooden floor for scrubbing.

Multi-level bristles look attractive because they reach different ins and outs of tooth rows, but their design follows the horizontal movement of the brush. I am propagating the differential "vertical" movement of the brush.

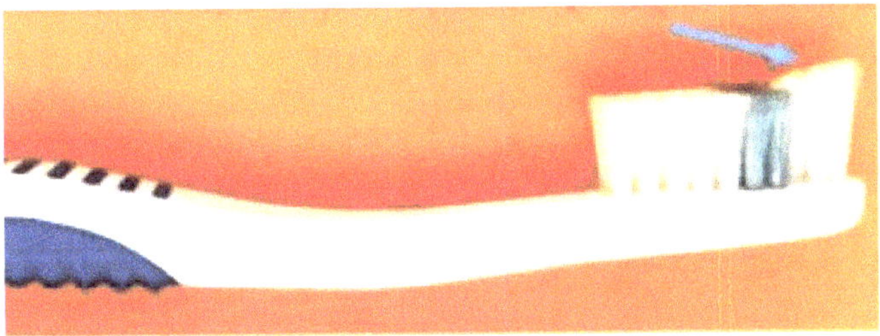

This sounds too apparent, but the convenience of the brush's handle in wet hands is important. In contrast with easy horizontal hand movement, the correct circular movements require some dexterity, training, and... convenience.

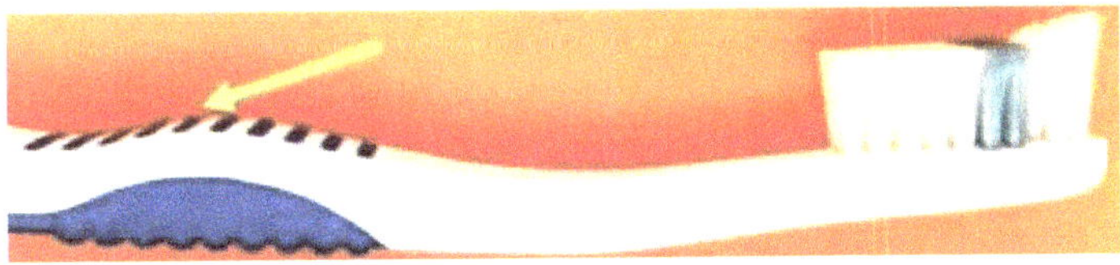

Tongue scrapers

This is the title of an article: *Tongue **scraping** for treating halitosis* (Cochrane Database Syst Rev. 2006). Similar articles exist.

In my view, tongue scraping definition is wrong. It determines the employment of inadequate tongue cleaning tools, not limited to fighting halitosis. They can be used occasionally, but the toothbrush should be the main tool for everyday routine.

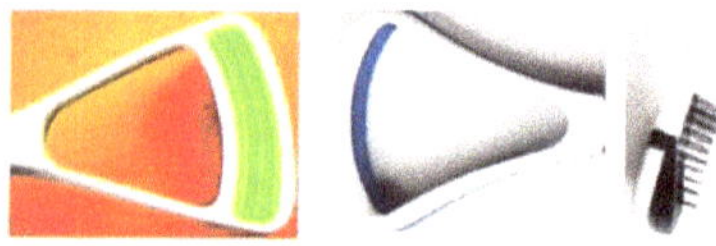

As an anatomic pathologist with a tongue in my hands and a histology picture in front of my eyes, I visualize a rigid scraper touching a different definition shape of the tongue while inevitably sliding above the tongue's papillae, where the microbiota hides (see the Anatomy section). The multiple different-shaped papillae are covered by thin, invisible microflora biofilm. Moreover, they can be damaging on some medical occasions because tongue scrapers are used without paste.

The goal is tongue cleaning with a toothbrush in which thin bristles deliver diluted paste to create a foamy environment between papillae for the expulsion of excessive products of microbial metabolism along with the perpetrators. It is neither scrapping a dirty floor nor patting a cat.

Powered toothbrush

Powered, electric, and sonic models of toothbrushes can be useful as gum massage devices. Their circulatory fast bristles move does not allow the user to make differential cleaning treatments as described in the previous paragraph. Moreover, the quick, difficult, manageable brush can inevitably "insert" some remnant of food into the gingival sulcus, where they would be trapped. A tooth is not a car in a carwash. There is an exception, however, when such a circular move could be used to clean premolars and molars cups.

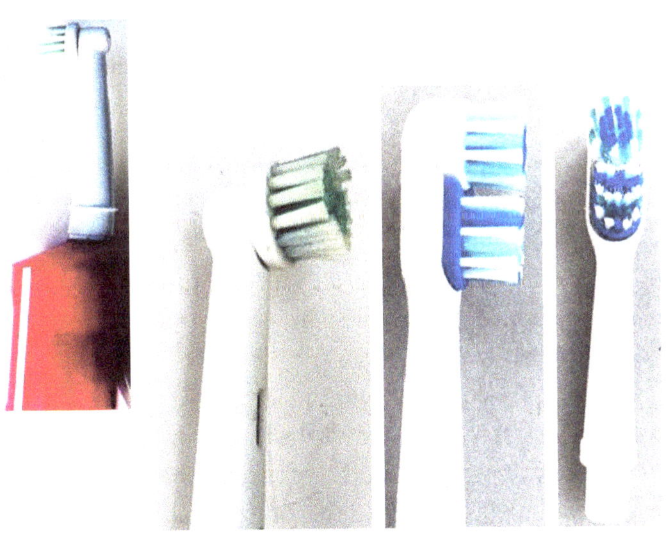

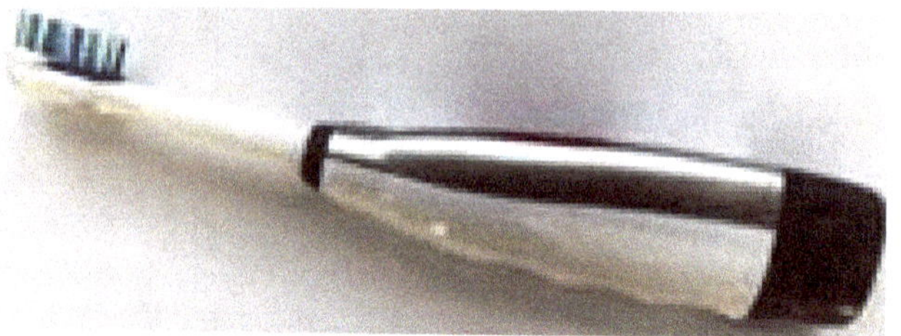

A powered toothbrush can be used for applications formulated especially for teeth pumice polishing.
Dental hygienists finish the cleaning procedure with this action, leaving a pleasant taste in the mouth of a flavoring agent when *Mint Flavored Professional Strength Tooth Polish* is applied. I would suggest intensive rinsing after using pumice at home to eliminate the gritty abrasive remnants.

I could not encounter credible studies that have found that electronic or powered toothbrushes may get rid of plaque better than manual toothbrushing. According to the American Dental Association:" *Either manual or powered toothbrushes can be used effectively."*

The article Krukovsky et al. *J Clin Dent* 2014; 25: 6-12 is an example of the ADA's approval references scientific base.
CONCLUSION The oscillating-rotating toothbrush demonstrated statistically significantly greater reductions in whole-mouth plaque at Weeks 6 and 12 and significantly greater gingivitis reductions over the long term (12 weeks), compared to the new sonic toothbrush. I do not understand the methodology of these studies, especially the plague scoring reduction. I have placed this reference here for readers' further exploration.

 Perhaps the following sentences are unnecessary, but just in case. The brush's vigorous rinse after every use is obligatory. The brush should be kept in a vertical position. Periodical baths and disinfection should be during its use.

A parenthetical remark

The conditions and appearance of people's teeth are signs of a civilized life. Teeth became a matter of esthetic, cosmetic, and personal psychological comfort. Dental offices advertise an attractive suggestion to "Keep Your Smile," although not every person's smile opens to show an excellent combination of teeth and gums. A massive billboard in Chicago reads: "I make sexy teeth." Parents spend money on teeth alignment to contribute, besides education, to their children's future careers, where the smile becomes a credential, supplanting the name of a prestigious university in a resume. The Invisalign brand of aligner is in teenagers' everyday vernacular.

As far as dental hygiene is concerned, tooth alignment can benefit more efficient tooth brushing by reaching every part of the dental arcade. Additionally, perhaps tooth alignment is beneficial in the prevention of enamel cracks, which, in the case of extremely hard food, can occur when the vertical power is not dispersed equally, especially due to simultaneous inherited tooth eruption and permanent tooth growth.

Toothpaste/Dentifrices

Introductory remarks

In contrast with toothbrushes, toothpaste is an area where I am still forming my understanding. The number of variants is impressive when you enter Walgreens or CVC stores. Is such abundance justified? My problem is that I do not have confidence in the research behind these variants.

Just one example without mentioning the product due to marketing consideration. A dentistry journal published a special issue devoted to studies on a toothpaste' type that allegedly has a bactericide ability. No, microbiology and morphology data are in all articles. A single image includes a line *"in the biofilm sagittal section* (sic!)", that leaves the impression that the authors of numerous articles do not understand the biofilm issue. Almost all authors of the articles worked at the manufacturing paste company. This is not nitpicking but a reflection of my impression of the research literature on toothpaste. A study paper without every detail of the methodology does not instill any trust in me. The reproductivity of the results is the main value of a study. These considerations form the basis of my attitude toward studies in dental hygiene.

According to the American Dental Association (ADA), there are three main types of toothpaste: Antimicrobial, Tartar control, and Whitening., ADA's classification does not provide specific ingredient support for this classification.

Antimicrobial paste

Antimicrobial pastes should include bactericide components. They are applied predominantly during toothbrushing. Let's return to one of brushing's goals: getting rid of dental plaques. This would inevitably be a partial repetition of previous materials in the *General Part*.

A plaque is formed by colonies aggregation of microorganisms embedded in a complex intercellular matrix of polymers on a tooth surface in a structurally organized soft, sticky, "thick" biofilm. Microorganisms form stable biofilms on many body surfaces, but a plague is referred to specifically on teeth.

Gradually, according to its own physiological rules, a plague is formed from a diversity of microorganisms to maintain microbial homeostasis. To some degree, a plague might protect against the intrusion of pathogenic microorganism species. Under certain conditions or too favorable a supply of carbohydrate sources for bacterial metabolism, the "guard" becomes overpopulated and requires downsizing.

A toothbrush is employed for downsizing plague biofilm pellicles' adhesion to the tooth surface. The antimicrobial chemical content can bring a new component to microbial homeostasis.

How far do we want to go?

A breakdown of the homeostatic mechanisms that normally maintain the relationship between the teeth and oral microflora can negatively affect periodontal disease, where gems, the pathogen bacteria, are the main damaging participants.

Clinical observations are not sufficient; experimental studies are necessary. Some brands state on the box that they "have not been tested on animals." In my view, understanding manufacturers' good intentions does not ensure quality.

The toothbrushing procedure is usually finished with more or less vigorous rinsing. The antibacterial component needs time for chemical reactions in the background of every disinfection process. It is not enough due to immediate rinsing. The potential antimicrobial effect is nullified by the spitting out rinsing water in sewage. I doubt the antimicrobial paste premise.

Tartar control paste

Dental calculus is a mineralized plaque on a tooth surface. It is a sequentially generated complex that entraps microbial, dietary, host, and ancient debris during spontaneous calcification events. It is composed primarily of calcium phosphate mineral salts deposited between and within remnants of formerly viable microorganisms and is covered by an unmineralized bacterial layer.

Dental calculus forms on the subgingival and/or supragingival tooth surfaces throughout an individual's life. It continues until it reaches a maximum, after which it may be reduced in amount or even broken due to its vulnerability. However, such supragingival tartar requires professional scaling with tooth protection, as in the photo below.

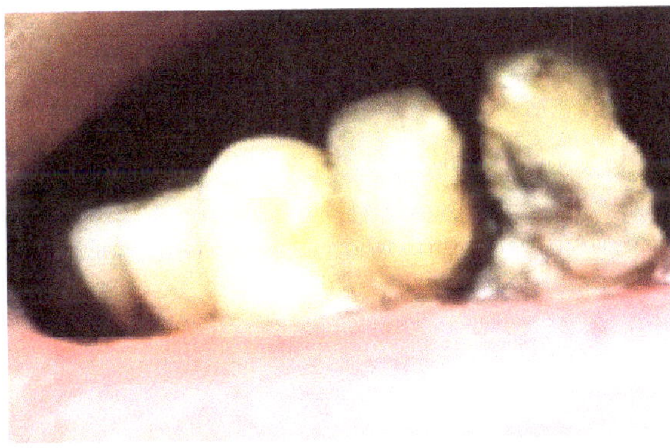

Excessive tartar formation on the canine tooth of the lower jaw.

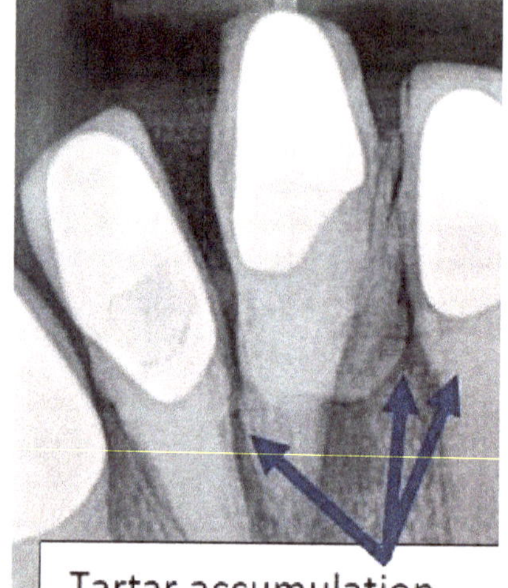

X-ray

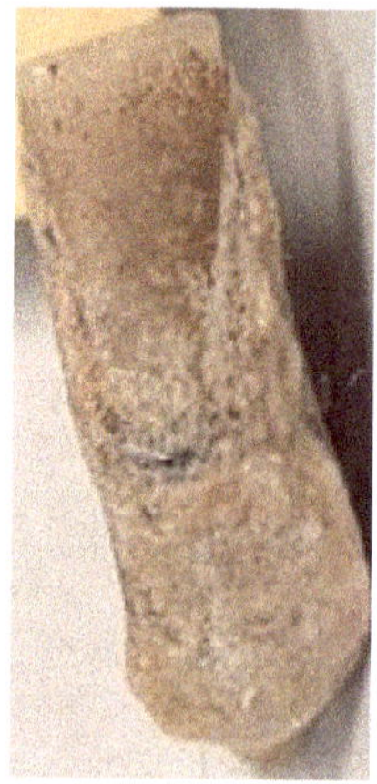

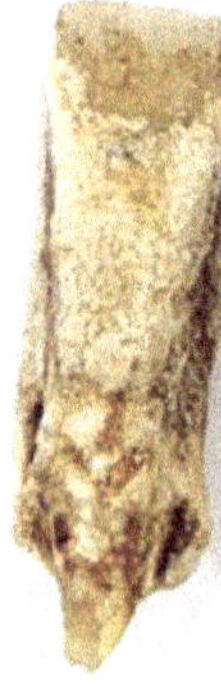
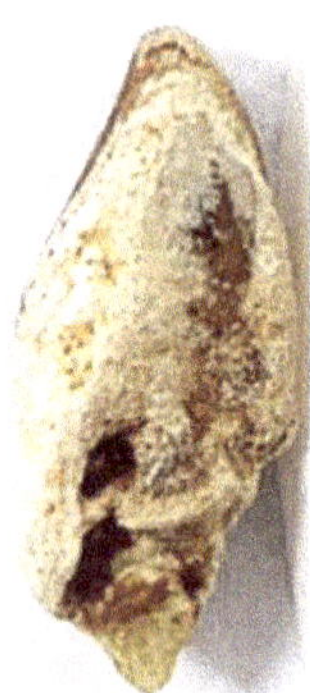

Evenly subgingival tartar

Patchy distribution of tartar

The more I dived into the literature, the more I realized that tartar formation mechanisms are still poorly understood. It is important for me to understand the procedure background by describing the chemical ingredients of the tartar control pastes. If the supragingival calculus can be somehow specifically managed by the individual's prophylactic care, the subgingival can be reached only by a professional hygienist.

Moreover, according to scientific studies, calculus's development is predominately of saliva's high pH which is the condition of mineralization by calcium and other minerals at the plagues that is completely opposite to demineralization of dentine, the main concern of caries prevention, as well as the enamel's damage. It comes to preventing the excessive microbial biofilm that is a plague. The rate of calculus accumulation varies among individuals and at different times in the same person. However, the regular standard dental hygiene procedures, which control excessive plaque formation are also a way of prevention, especially among so-called heavy calculus formers.

Most implants do not accumulate much calculus buildup unless they are in the lower front jaw area.

Microorganisms are not always essential in calculus formation because calculus occurs readily in germ-free rodents.

Whitening paste

While essentially cosmetic, this group of pastes is also inevitably part of dental hygiene. No paste does not mention whitening. The tooth color depends on the enamel's thickness and the dentin's color. A plague, actually a biofilm, is translucent unless it is not becoming tartar, which accumulates other substances. White teeth are not healthier than teeth with a yellowish color. However, the white color indirectly is evidence that teeth care takes place and is more attractive.

I believe whitening at the expense of thin translucent enamel would not be correct. Calk is suitable for whitening, but it is too abrasive for enamel. As mentioned, whitening paste should differ from regular everyday teeth cleaning patterns. The brush's movements are horizontal by hand or circular by power brush. No rinsing is expected, like after a polish paste with mint flavor in the dental office.

Again, prophylactic dental hygiene toothbrushing and whitening are different procedures. For whitening, the procedure should be called paste application. Manufacturers should appropriately instruct users of paste, which is declared to be whitening.

Salt toothpastes. I do not know about the polishing effect of such pastes, like Zesty Sea salt. The amount of salt and time of application are not enough to have an osmotic hypertonic impact. As participants in standard dental hygiene routines, they are useless.

Toothpaste ingredients

I am stepping into a very unclear zone of issues that must be addressed. I'm not going to discuss brands or provide any recommendations for them.

Active ingredient

My "classification" of all toothpastes would divide them into two groups: with Sodium fluoride or without it. Most of them include fluoride (0,243%, rarely 0.454%), which is an active ingredient. Only a few brands are declaring "Nonfluoride" on the market.

Active ingredient   **Purposes**
Stannous fluoride 0.454% (0.15% w/v fluoride ion)........................Anticavity, Antigingivitis, Antihypersensitivity

or

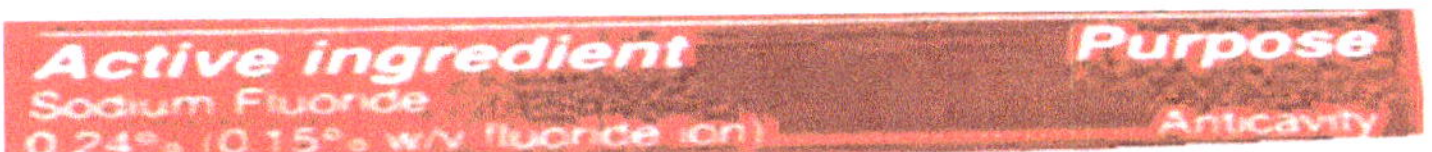

It is common knowledge that fluoride is a component of enamel formation and durability. This is why fluoride salts are added to drinking water or consumed differently. In this situation, it is incorporated into the person's metabolism as a component.

When Sodium fluoride is applied in a paste during toothbrushing, there is not enough time for a chemical reaction because the salt is diluted by saliva and spilled out after rinsing. Some chemicals work instantly on an appropriate substance, but this is not the case for Sodium fluoride in such a concentration as a paste with the following rinsing under toothbrushing conditions.

This brings us to the question of whether to rinse or not to rinse after brushing.

My point is that any chemical reaction requires time of duration, in contrast to osmotic action, which works just at the moment of application. I cannot understand how Sodium fluoride even penetrates the plague for its bactericide abilities, as some studies claim. When I jumped into the fluoride literature, I encountered reviews with references on reviews, which referenced studies without details on the methodology that, for me, was utterly worthless. I will continue to search for credible sources. At this time, I only express my doubts. I would be glad to encounter credible studies, especially with morphology verification. However, the latter is challenging to achieve due to reasons that I mentioned already in the Introduction to *Methods and Tools* section.

As mentioned in the brushing section, rinsing after paste application is rational. If some paste traces remain on the teeth' surface, let them do the work the paste is applied to do.

Inactive ingredients

The rest of the paste's content is called inactive ingredients. They are numerous and very similar in different brands. I doubt that they are read or that their purpose is understood.

The so-called inactive ingredients are a fascinating group with mysterious names, such as Mica. Thanks to the ingredients list, I discovered this is a skincare silicate mineral.

So-called inactive ingredients determine the difference between pastes. Most importantly, they make the paste work or not.

The examples of inactive ingredients are below. It isn't easy to distinguish them in different brands.

Inactive ingredients water, hydrated silica, sorbitol, glycerin, PEG-8, cocamidopropyl betaine, flavor, titanium dioxide, xanthan gum, sodium saccharin, sodium hydroxide

or

Inactive Ingredients Water, Sorbitol, Hydrated Silica, PEG-12, Sodium Lauryl Sulfate, Flavor, Cellulose Gum, Potassium Hydroxide, Tetrasodium Pyrophosphate, Phosphoric Acid, Cocamidopropyl Betaine, Sodium Saccharin

Usually, it is unclear why they are participants in the paste, but one brand accompanied the list of inactive ingredients with explanations of why these chemicals are in the paste. I want to present it to readers who would find similar names on their brands.

Just from the box (in italics): *"Sorbitol (humectant) purified water, hydrated silica (polishes and clean teeth).vegetable glycerin (moisturizes), calcium carbonate (polishes and cleans teeth, xylitol (sweetener), erythritol (sweetener), xanthan gum (thickener) flavor (freshens breath), titanium dioxide (appearance), cocos nucifera (coconut)oil (moisturizes), zinc citrate (controls tartar), cocamidopropyl betaine (cleanser) sodium cocoyl glutamate (cleanser), potassium sorbate (maintains stability), steve rebaudiana leaf extract (sweetener) and melaleuca alternifolia (tea tree) leafoil (cleans and freshens breath).* No my comment, but I 've read the list with an interest.

Most of these ingredients are included in different brands of pastes. I'm not going to discuss them and the differences between brands. I intentionally do not mention any brand.

One thing would be reasonable, in my view, to remark. Although people become adherent to certain brands for many reasons, I would suggest that perhaps it is not right. The ingredients are a little bit different. They do not have direct bactericide effects but might be preferable for certain types of microorganisms, which become prevalent and lead to their ability to build biofilms and plagues. We are interested in natural selection in the microbiota that limits the expansion of one of the groups. *"They (bacteria) killing each other like crazy"* exclaimed once a microbiology scientist.

It is just a suggestion by a pathologist who respects the laws of evolution to change periodically a brand of the paste., because the brand is more a personal preference of the taste. I interviewed many people, including at the store shelves and my surrounding during this book preparation.

To conclude my remarks on toothpaste, I want to underline that all pastes, independently of their brands, should be used as facilitators for toothbrushing to eliminate food remnants and make the microbial biofilms plague.

For this purpose, the paste should be able to generate foam for adequate rinsing. There is no substantial difference between washing hands and doing laundry. These details are discussed in the current book's Standard Tooth Brushing Pattern section at the end of the Special Part.

What kind of paste would I prefer? I would use the **foamiest** to others.

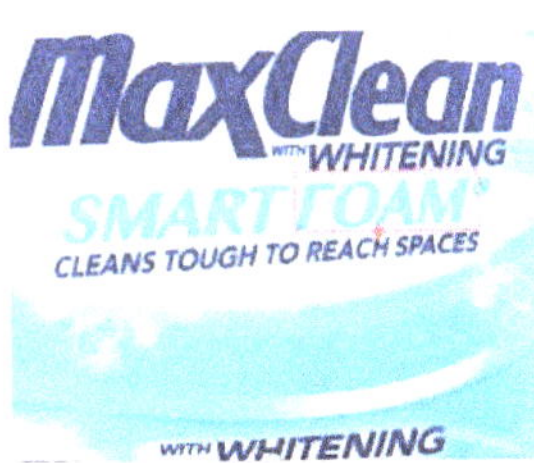

The taste, smell, and convenience of tube handling (opening the cap) are personal preferences. I do not want to touch the price issue. However, in my believe the price of the paste is not necessarily important and reflects the quality, as I experimented with many brands.

Toothbrushing powders

The old-fashioned teeth cleaning powder remains used, but the American Dental Association hasn't accepted it.

 Over 90% of the ingredients are chemically precipitated chalk, sometimes white bentonite clay and activated charcoal. There are even homemade tooth powders.

There are recommendations for occasionally brushing teeth with baking soda for a deeper clean. For example, I've read: "You just sprinkle it on your toothbrush with water and scrub your teeth. It does help to give you that squeaky-clean feeling. Because baking soda is abrasive, you don't want to do this more than once a week."

A study claimed that toothpaste is statistically superior to toothpaste in controlling dental plaque and gingivitis (*Compend Contin Educ Dent*. 2017 Sep;38(8): e13-e1).

Despite all the positive ingredients that can be added to the powder, it does not provide a foamy environment at the end of brushing, which is essential during rinsing to remove food remnants from the teeth.

In general, the powder is abrasive, although is used for whitening.

Flossing/ Interdental cleaning

The definition of dental flossing is more than 150 years old. This action is apparent and rational because it gets gunk between the teeth to prevent tooth decay. In essence, it is interdental cleaning, defined as flossing because the instrument for it, floss (soft thread), was patented for this purpose in the mid-19th century. This terminological clarification is necessary because it brings common sense to this dental hygiene action.

The American Dental Association (ADA) recommends flossing once daily for teeth. I will not discuss the presence of compelling studies supporting the recommendation. In the same line, I don't want even to argue numerous used on occasions substitutes to clear the spaces between teeth as fingernails, folded paper, forks, safety pins, and others. . I insist that flossing should be considered at the level of a medical procedure with its main adage: *Do not harm*.

What

The dental hygiene literature sets the goal of flossing to reduce plaque and stuff caught between the teeth. I would place the second as the first. The main goal is to eliminate remnants of carbohydrate-type food, more specifically, minute crumbs. Concerning reducing plaque, the actual flossing technique is not indisputably beneficial.

How

The working floss is usually recommended to be 18 inches (45 cm) long and sometimes applied with a threader. I'm not going to provide instructions on flossing techniques, but I want to comment directly on some descriptions that I've picked up from different sources.

*"Hold the floss tightly between the thumbs and forefingers and **gently** insert it between the teeth. Curve the floss into a 'C' shape against the side of the tooth." "Do not snap the floss between teeth. Instead, **gently** slide 'back and forth' on the sides of each tooth in a **gentle** 'lasso' by rubbing the floss along the sides of the teeth before gently removing the floss through the contact of the two teeth." "**Gently** slide the floss down towards the gum margins of each tooth and when finished cleaning the sides of the teeth, simply pull the floss straight out and do not pull back up towards the top of the tooth called the marginal ridge." "Press the floss into your gumline, form it into a C-shape, and run it **gently** up and down the sides of both teeth."*

I placed the word *gently* in bold because it was right. It reflects the sole purpose of the procedure: to remove remnants of food rather than plagues that require pressure. Concerning reducing plaque, the actual flossing technique is not indisputably beneficial.

Another quote: "Now for what I learned in dental school. I was taught that for flossing to be effective; you have to adapt the floss to the interproximal surfaces of the teeth and floss down **subgingival** 5-7x on each surface." Besides 5-7x, which is rarely used, the word **subgingival** in bold is important. In this situation, the floss is touching the most vulnerable area as the gingival sulcus.

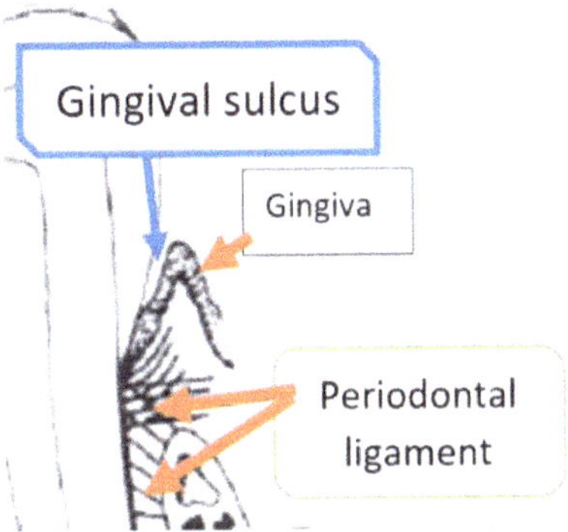

The diagram presents an excerpt from the tooth diagram in the section devoted to the periodontal ligament, pointing to the critical place—the gingival sulcus—where the traditional flossing technique could reach. It is a narrow space between the gingiva and the tooth covered by thin junctional epithelium. Inevitably, the epithelium is stripped away. The pocket-like space becomes a collection of tissue debris, remnants of food, and some blood components, even if blood is not visible (epithelium does not have vessels). The microbiota balance is disrupted. The excess of "ingredients" for bacterial metabolism provides a nutritional feast for benign or even pathological germs.

In conclusion

I suggest that people can do traditional flossing with some degree of skill after some training. It is essential to avoid damaging the gum papilla. Too vigorous flossing might cause mini cracks in the enamel.

It isn't easy to floss the entire tooth. If the thread is placed at the gum level, the subgingival thread movements on the circa of the tooth can cause more harm than good.

To floss before or after tooth brushing?

Flossing does not substitute for tooth brushing; it follows tooth brushing. It is optimal, but there could be exceptions for convenience reasons.

In my view, flossing is a final assault on food remnants. It is an addition to tooth brushing, with no attempt to go for the plaque. But really, when a person is in the mood to do this tedious procedure.

Flossing "quality control" tests suggestions

The presented "quality control test is just my suggestion. They can be implemented in routine dental hygiene practices.

Odor "test"

Perhaps this sounds unpleasant and weird, but a floss thread or an interdental brush should be periodically sniffed after being removed from the mouth. Rotting food spoilage odors can indicate that the interdental space was not cleaned properly. Such a test would be most appropriate after flossing under the dental bridges.

Iodine–starch test

Remembering my old work with blood and urine amylase tests, I suggest a floss thread impingent with iodine can be used as a test for clearing the interdental space and even other areas from remnants of starch-containing food. The dental microflora metabolism uses starch as the main substrate.

Upon contact with starch, the triiodide anion instantly produces an intense blue-black color. The stain can be detected visually even when the concentration of the iodine and starch is low. This is an old test that was used in the food industry. Of course, such a test requires some experimentation before suggesting for practice.

With

Interdental cleaning/flossing generally includes three main devices: classic string floss (Dental floss)/dental picks, interdental tiny brushes, or water picks/flossers.

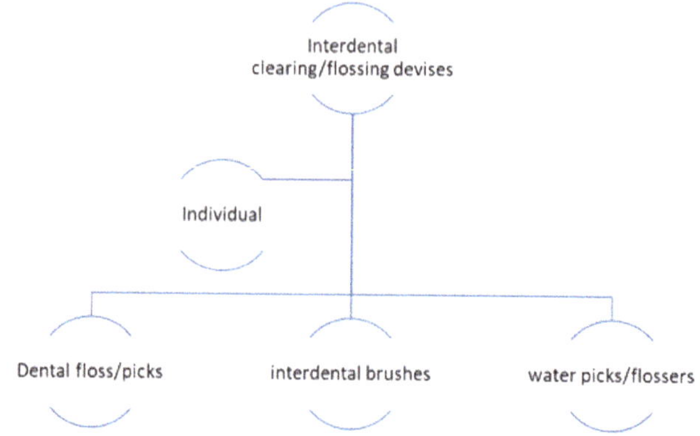

Dental floss has a regular floss thread, spongy floss, and a threader with a stiffened end. It includes different types of strings (waxed-unwaxed, synthetic -Polytetrafluoroethylene, braided nylon; wider, flatter, or variable diameter). I'm not going to discuss the advantages of each because each is individual and should be customized by the hygienist.

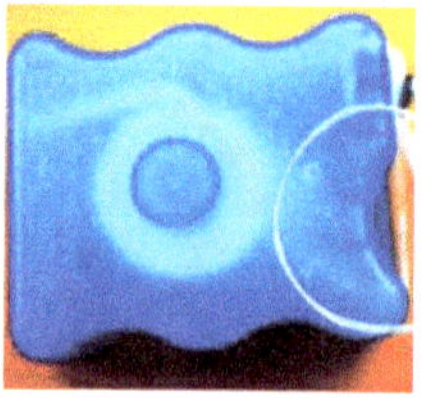

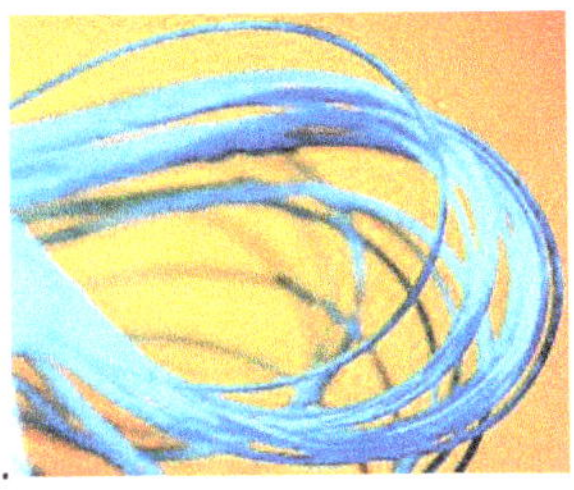

Dental floss threader   Dental floss threader's loop (eye)

I don't doubt that despite my critical remarks regarding traditional flossing with a smooth strand of nylon or Teflon, it will be used for a forcible future. Dental floss can reach the tiny crevices between teeth that a toothbrush can't.

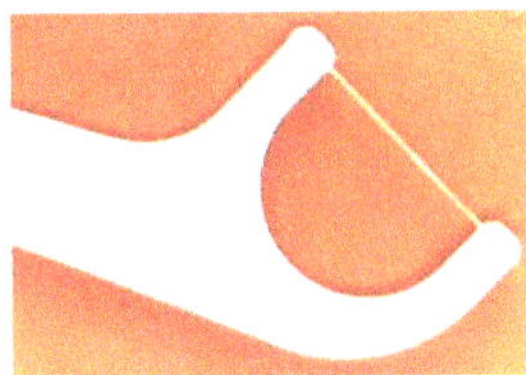

Floss picks consist of a small handle with two end posts holding a short floss string. Also referred to as floss sticks, they can be used as an alternative to a wooden toothpick.

Traditional flossing does not have a good perspective. It cannot clean areas under braces, retainers, and bridges.

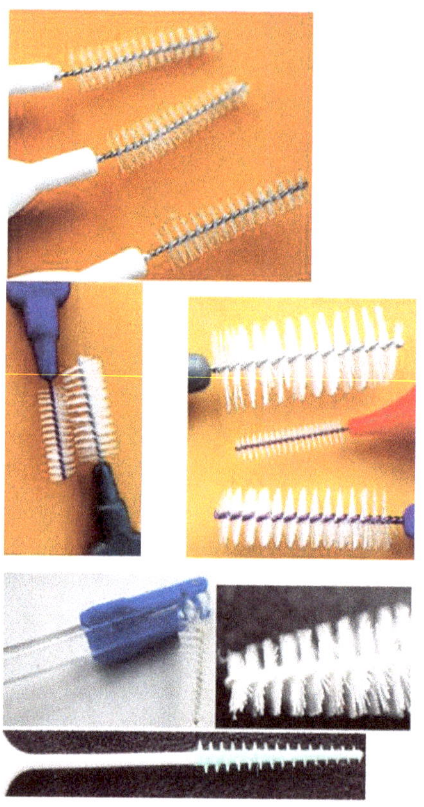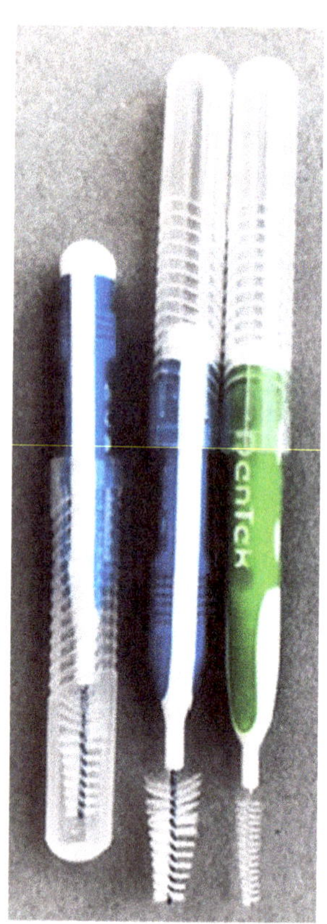

Interdental brushes with different sizes of tiny nylon bristles reach spaces not covered by gingival papillae. Perhaps the variety of interdental brushes presented reflects my bias toward them. This positive attitude is determined by their convenience and the minimal possibility of traumatizing the gums.

Interdental brushes require intensive rinsing under a stream of tap water after use in every space between teeth. They should be kept in a disinfection solution.

Plastic interdental picks are distributed by a dentist to patients. They can be used only if something stock that cannot be taken out by other tools.

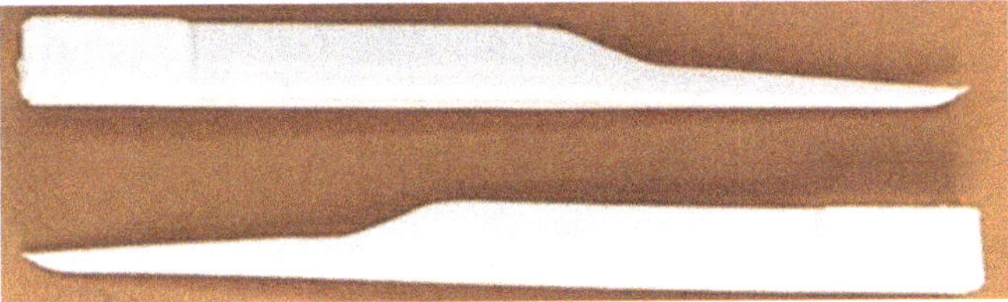

Dental scalers are entirely unacceptable for personal prophylactic dental hygiene. They can be traumatic, and their effectiveness in removing plaque and tartar is questionable. Scaling should be left to professional dental hygienists.

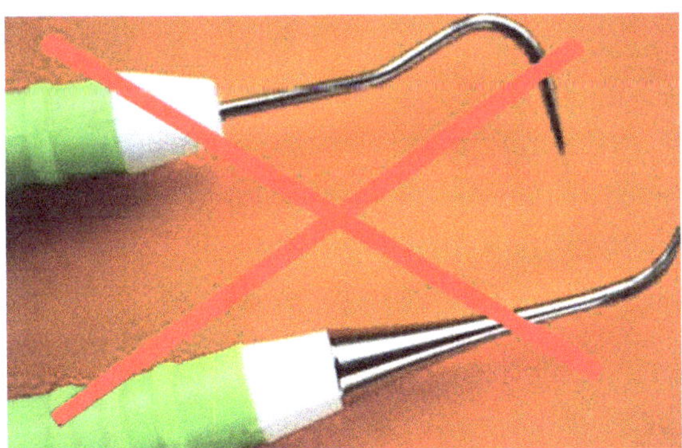

And now comes the heavyweight in play, the water pick. It resembles a power wash. While a power brush can be negative in some occasions, a water pick does not have any negatives except the cost and propensity for misfunctioning. People with braces, bridges, and other dental work may find that a water flosser helps them reach everywhere (nook and cranny).

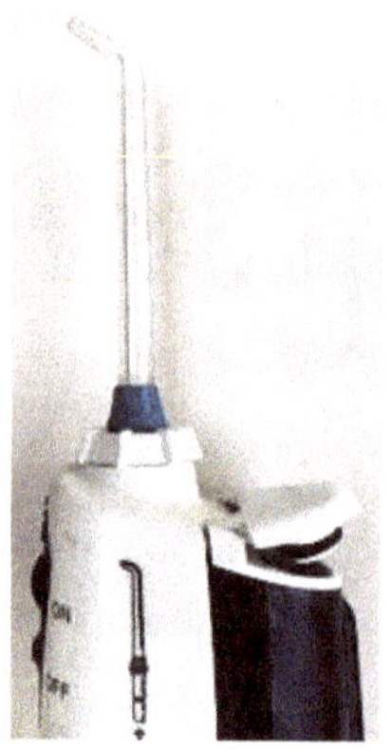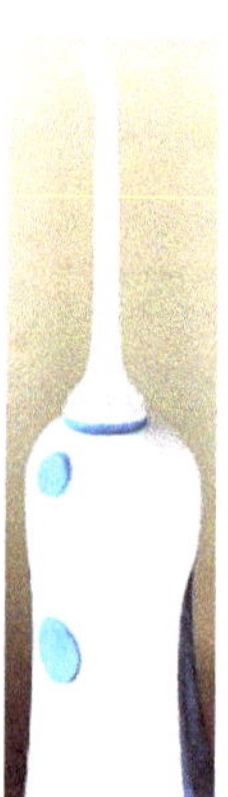

Different types of power water flossers, sophisticated with warm pulsating water or simple cordless. They intend to deliver an effective clean of all areas of the mouth, including hard-to-reach areas like back teeth and even a little under the gumline. They are especially efficient in the case of different sizes of bridges when the brush apparently cannot reach the area between the gum and the bridge, while flossing requires some skills and time to insert the flossing tread under the bridge.

In summary

I am ambivalent about the preferred flossing method. A toothbrush is just a brush, but many interdental cleaning options exist. Below is a summary of my considerations.

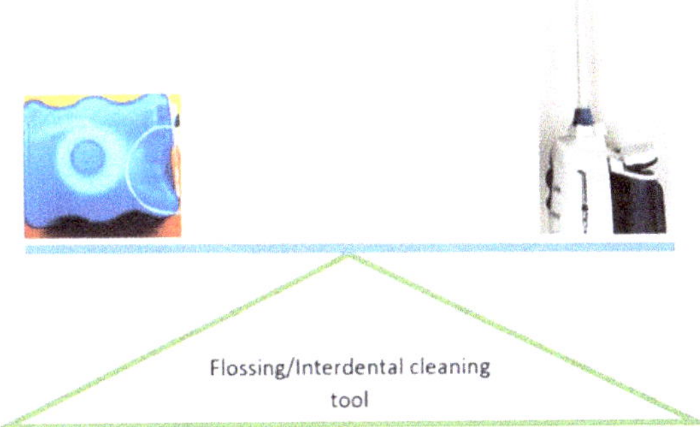

I consider the method primarily because it could violate the first principle of medicine: not to harm.

 This depends on many factors, but the main one is the dexterity/skill of the person doing the flossing. Effective flossing is also determined by the time allocated, diligence, and numerous other aspects of a particular person's circumstances. And cost cannot be out of the choice. The Waterpik device has an advantage if these conditions cannot be met positively. The Waterpik device is preferable for dental work under the conditions mentioned above. Of course, both can be used, but I referred to the preference. On many occasions, both might be used. As mentioned above, I prefer interdental brushes, including for personal reasons.

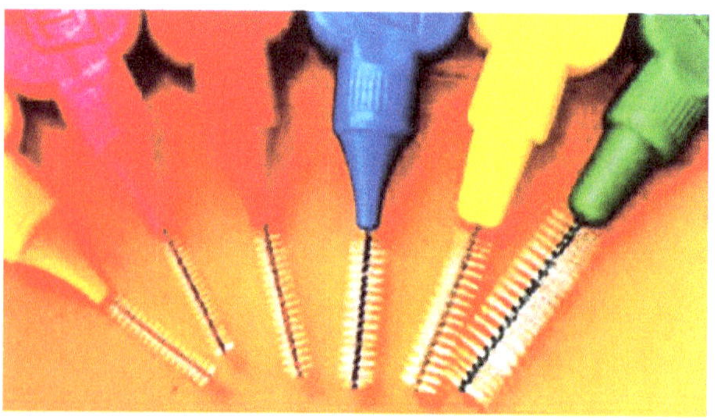

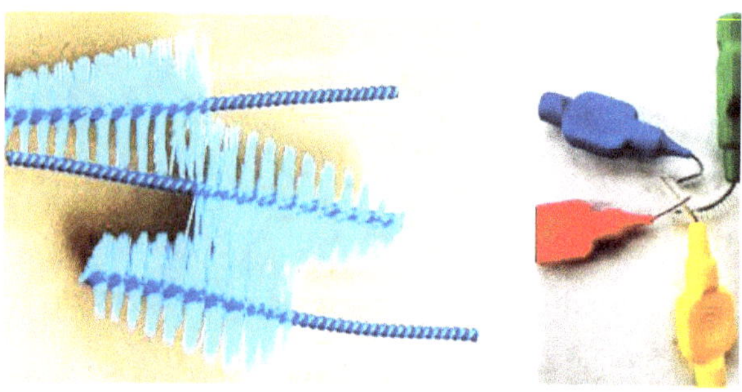

Again, interdental cleaning devices should be customized according to personal circumstances due to the different spaces between teeth. Brushes are available in different width sizes and are bendable, which is sometimes necessary to reach the back of the teeth or a single tooth. When doing dishes, something goes in the dishwasher, and something is done by hand. It depends. And again, if after sniffing an interdental brush, a person smells an unpleasant odor, this means that it is necessary to return to the everyday dental hygiene procedure.

Rinsing

Some introductory words

I want to provide a disclaimer before presenting the rinsing material in my standard WHAT, HOW, AND WITH pattern.

I understand that many things might sound like travesties, but I hope the potential reader will have some sense of humor and share this understanding with me. My professional attitude towards details might also influence the narrative.

Rinsing has an apparent physical component. It is predominant. Mechanical vibration, partial osmosis diffusion, and momentary soaking vacuum gradient are in the background of the physical component.

The chemical component is beyond my understanding, and the time duration allocated for chemical reactions is minimal.

What/Why

The "theoretical" background for rinsing is already presented in the previous sections about teeth brushing and flossing. I'm repeating the premise that the main aim of prophylactic oral hygiene is to prevent the microbiota/microflora/bacteria inhabitants from consuming food leftovers for their metabolism.

An additional outcome of rinsing can be what dental literature euphemistically calls cosmetic, but in reality, it is to eliminate unpleasant feelings in the mouth and potentially malodor. The latter is predominately apparent in the mornings because saliva secretion is diminished during sleep, and the final products of the microorganism's metabolism are retained in the mouth.

Under certain conditions, rinsing can help reduce plaque after teeth brushing and flossing. However, the outcome should not be overestimated. I have definite reservations about rinsing as a direct teeth/mouth disinfection action.

Obviously, rinsing action depends on time, purpose, type of rinse, and individual preferences. I'll discuss in some detail water rinsing. Repetitions are also inevitable because the entire process is artificially divided for the sake of concentration on details.

How

Short rinsing is reasonable before both procedures because some remnants, especially minute crumbs, can be accidentally placed in the subgingival area, especially the gingival sulcus, and it would be difficult to remove them from there. An energetic rinse after these procedures, especially brushing, is obligatory to help the foamy paste finish the job.

Some recommendations are to hold the paste for a while in the mouth after brushing by leaving the fluoride from the toothpaste for a longer time for a better effect. This is wrong because all gunk taken away from the teeth during brushing is left in the mouth. The amount of saliva increases, which requires inevitable swallowing. And how long would it be before rinsing? Brushing is not our goal in life. It is done and forgotten.

Fluoride dentification should be a particular procedure according to prescription unrelated to standard tooth brushing, and this is a different story, which I've already discussed in the toothpaste section. Or, you can apply a pea-sized amount of toothpaste like a medical treatment but, again, not a regular tooth brushing procedure.

Cold or warm water depends not only on personal preferences and tolerance. Usually, it does not matter. Cold water is obligatory if brushing or flossing generates even traces of bleeding. Bacteria will appreciate the substrate of blood proteins after the procedure. However, better warm water is in every laundry process. About the latter later below.

When In my belief, water rinsing should be carried out immediately after a meal, which is rarely achievable and questionably desirable unless the meal is ugly. However, from the ideal point of dental hygiene, a mouth empty of remnants of food can be achieved only by maximally following the end of any food intake.

With

According to the American Dental Association (ADA), there are two main types of mouthwash (also called mouthwash): cosmetic and therapeutic. In modern life, three main rinsing "devices" might participate in individual dental hygiene in their varieties: water, mouthwash, and special medically targeted mouthwash.

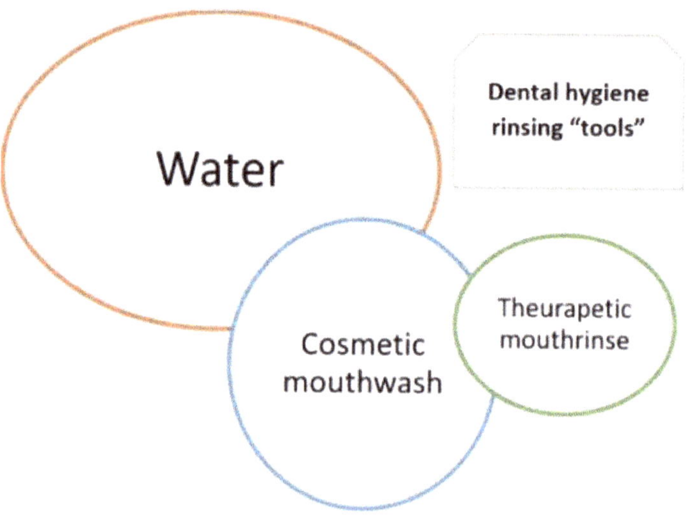

In the diagram, water, cosmetic mouthwash, and therapeutic mouth rinse are placed in different circles to distinguish them by their purpose. The size of the circles reflects my attitude toward all three.

Water

Again, avoiding sliding is a travesty, so I want to defend my preference for water and touch on some details. All my statements in this regard are biased.

Tap or bottled water for rinsing might be a matter of discussion, and the opinions are so complicated and diverse that I do not want to touch them. In my view, tap water, unless unavailable in some situations, has a preference due to the unlimited amount available for this occasion in most areas of the USA, except in some cases guaranteed quality. Fluoride is added. There might be many exceptions in local areas or single-home water supply.

Cold or warm water depends not only on personal preferences and tolerance. Usually, it does not matter. Cold water is obligatory if brushing or flossing generates even traces of bleeding. Bacteria will appreciate the substrate of blood proteins after the procedure. However, warm water is needed for every laundry process.

The amount of water during every rinse does matter. It only looks that the more the better. In my view, just the opposite is right. Vigorous swishing is provided by buccal muscle movements which a full mouth of water can restrict. Salivatory glands are irritated and extra saliva is diluting the foamy content left after paste application. Finally, the person is urged to swallow part of the rinse bringing to the gut completely undesirable content.

Cosmetic mouthwash

Commonly, cosmetics are products or actions applied to an object to improve its appearance. In this context, I am referring to comfort mouthwashes—the less misleading the euphemism, the more meaningful the information about dental hygiene benefits.

According to the American Dental Association (ADA):" *Cosmetic mouth rinse may temporarily control bad breath and leave behind a pleasant taste, but have no chemical or biological application beyond their temporary benefi*t."

Unfortunately, a person can't control the foul smell or even feel it. Cosmetic mouthwashes, like perfume, fight the unpleasant taste in the mouth. More details are in the *Reflections on halitosis related to dental hygiene* entry on page 135 in the Appendices. Just a remark. Foul morning breath could be connected with low acidity of secretion in the stomach, especially after meat consumption when mouthwashes cannot be helpful.

Regarding other benefits, we have to rely on representative studies behind the features on the label. The ingredients cannot be completely indifferent, hopefully for good.

The industry manufactures different sizes of bottles. It would not be a bad idea to have a small one with a cup in your car.

Therapeutic mouth rinse

Being lost in variants on the market (enamel care, advanced multi-protection, bacteria guard, antiseptic oral rinse, etc.), I do not have any opinion regarding therapeutic mouth rinses for many reasons, including that I do not understand the methodological background of studies which support their usefulness.

Joseph Lister, the British surgeon, changed how the surgery was done by suggesting sterilization in the late 1800's. However, while keeping the surgery field and the operating room sterile as much as possible, we don't think our dental hygiene field should be kept sterile.

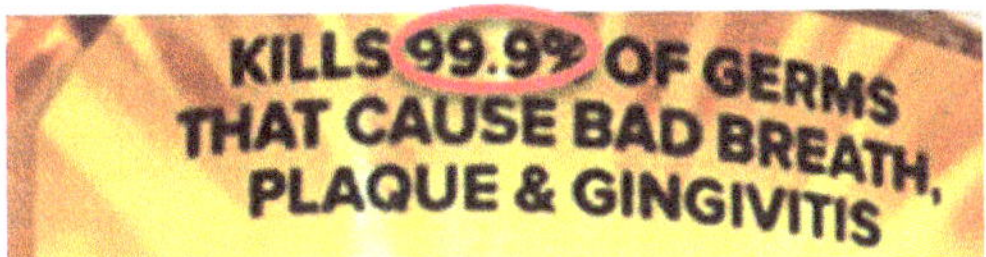

A sense of humor is a virtue.

 Different therapeutic mouth rinses include the same active and inactive ingredients, such as Eucalyptol, Mint, Methyl Salicylate, and Cetylpyridinium Chloride. If the concentration is so low that they are inactive, why place them in the solution or even mention them?

The rinse that falls in the medication category should be prescribed appropriately. This brings me to PerioGard.

PerioGard

Chlorhexidine Gluconate 0.12% (the generic for Peridex, PerioGard) is a mouthrinse. The pharmacies call it a Mouth/Throat solution. This is misleading. It should be distinguished from a regular therapeutic mouthrinse.

A dentist prescribes chlorhexidine for a special occasion (gingivitis, for instance) in a 15 ml (1/2 ounce, three tablespoons) dosage.

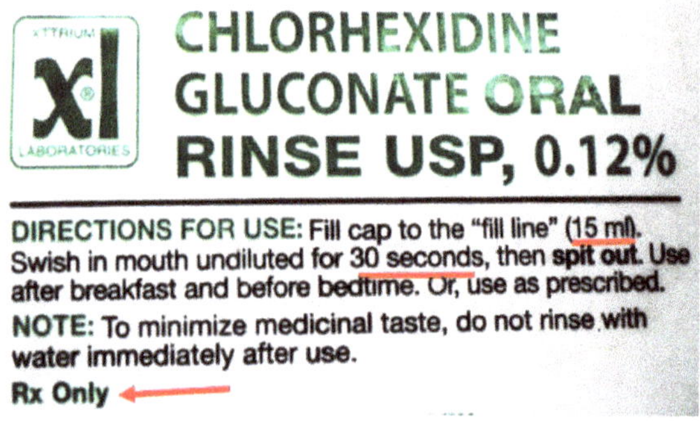

For orientation, three tablespoons are 15 ml and one drink is almost 30 ml. A regular sip is just 15 ml.

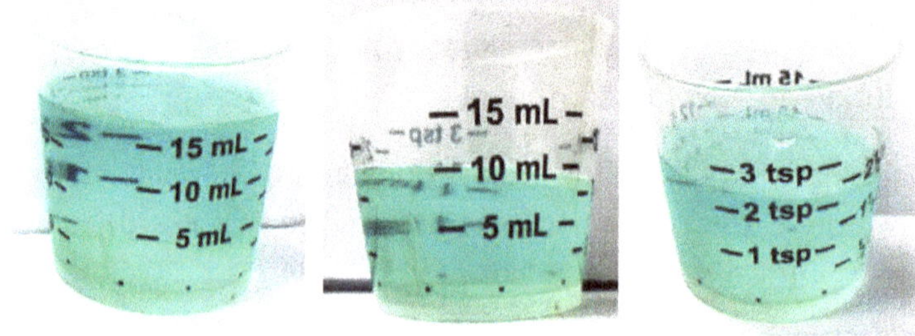

Again, PerioGard is not a rinse but a medication that should be treated appropriately. This is why the detailed suggestions below are included.

The dose can be less than 15 ml (two tablespoons), just enough to make some swishes. Keep it in the mouth as long as possible before spitting it out, as saliva will inevitably dilute the medication. Two spoons are better just for keeping the medication in the mouth longer.

I would suggest two-tablespoon increments (5 ml). This medication is not for entire-mouth irrigation but should be kept on the lower floor of the mouth, where the target of action is located in most cases. The upper jaw requires a different method, which requires more swishing with a minimal amount of the PerioGard.

After a minimal dose, no vigorous swish reaches the upper teeth arch. Tasting-like swishing movements by lips will reach the upper arcade just to wet it. Then, hold on at the lower jaw as long as tolerated before the urge to swallow. Then, energetic swish before spitting out. There is no swishing between them because it increases the saliva dilution of the medication.

Some dentists recommend even diluted PerioGard for sensitive mouth mucosa. The note on the bottle states: To minimize medicinal taste, do not rinse with water immediately after use.

I would suggest that you do not rinse at all as much as the taste is tolerated. No food or drink after. The final accord of food and drink consumption is over for today. See on page 108 PerioGard's use of periodontitis or other complications prevention in an "ill" tooth/teeth case.

With the same amount of used mouthwash (15 ml), the cosmetic mouthwashes generated more foam than the therapeutic, with a" cap" of bubbles above the cup while lingering for a longer time inside.

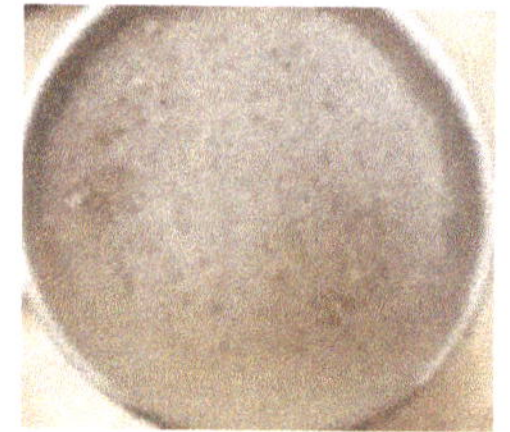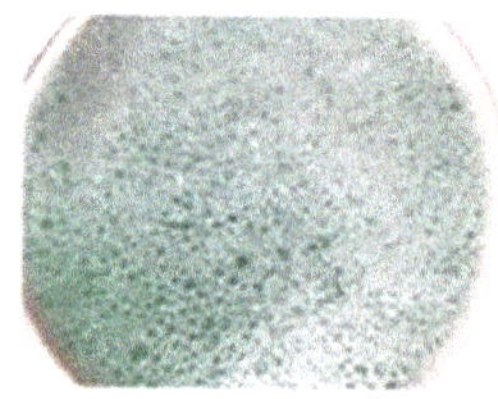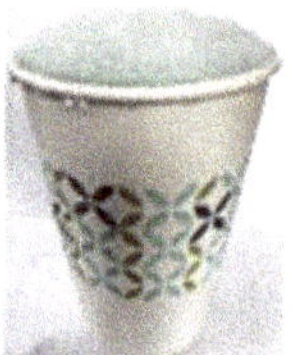

Therapeutic mouthwash   Cosmetic mouthwash

For therapeutic mouthwashes, the foamy content provides more penetration into targeted surfaces. Active and inactive ingredients provide the osmotic effect, which only works when minimal contact is made with targeted surfaces during rinsing.

(Some physics on water surface tension phenomena in Appendices entry Mouthwash foam formation physics, pages 158-164).

Alcohol in mouthwashes

One of the components in mouthrinse, which is widely discussed, is alcohol. I want to address this issue from my perspective.

First, ethanol alcohol is not acidic, as is sometimes stated. The pH value of alcohol is 7.33. It is neutral, like water. Aromatic alcohols could be slightly acidic but are not used in mouthrinse—the concentration of alcohol in mouthrinse ranges from 14% to 27%. For example, the Listerine brand contains 26.9%, Scope – 18.9%, and Cepacol – 14% alcohol. Beers contain 3-8% alcohol; wine contains 7-18%; spirits contain 30% or greater.

It's common knowledge that alcohol can kill bacteria. For example, it's commonly used as a disinfectant when blood is drawn. The disinfecting alcohol is 70-99% alcohol. However, alcohol is not added as a disinfectant in mouthrinse but rather as a carrier agent for active ingredients like four essential oils: eucalyptol, menthol, methyl salicylate, and thymol. in Listerine, and other chemicals according to recipes of a particular brand. The idea is to penetrate plagues. Or it is used as a preservative.

However, alcohol, as a drying mouth issue after using alcohol-containing mouthrinse, cannot be dismissed. Some sensitive people complain that they feel dry mouth. This might be a reason.

In this regard, I want to make an analogy with a histology laboratory tissue processing to get a paraffin microslide. A set of increased-concentration alcohols is used for tissue dehydration to insert paraffin into tissue. Alcohol makes lipoproteins more soluble for paraffin penetration. The exact mechanism would be close to the mouth mucous epithelium.

Salivary glands and dry mouth issues

While for the main salivary glands (parotid, submandibular, and sublingual) with long ducts, the low alcohol concentration is not significant, but for numerous, up to hundreds of so-called minor salivary glands of people with sensitive mouth mucosa, such alcohol irritation might be temporally damaging. In minor salivary glands, the secretory and excretory parts are very close; no ducts exist.

The salivary glands secretion is under complicated Autonomic nervous system (Vegetative nervous system), which includes the Sympathetic nervous system and Parasympathetic nervous system. The first restricts secretion (dry mouth under extreme stress, for example), and the second increases secretion (nighttime salivation, for example). I'm mentioning this without going into unrelated dental hygiene details only to prevent from jumping into *Post Hoc, Ergo Propter Hoc* (after this, therefore because of this) the drying mouth after using some alcohol-containing mouthrinse conclusions.

 In conclusion, the *Methods and Tools* Part, artificially separated for detailed discussion, must be underlined that toothbrushing, interdental cleaning/flossing, and rinsing work in concert. They are combined in the diagram by inseparable interactions, where the laws of physics and chemistry must be applied.

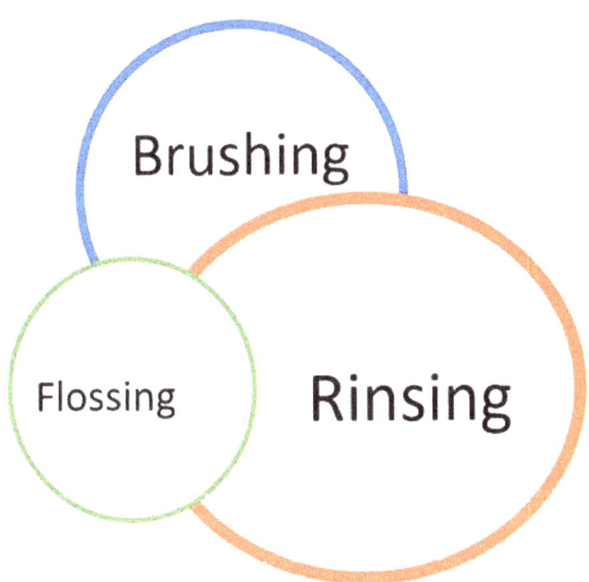

The Venn diagram circles are different sizes, reflecting my attitude toward these actions. My preference is determined by the level of precise mechanical actions and their intensity. However, this is a matter of my opinion.

Daily dental hygiene

This section presents approximate daily dental hygiene procedures for an average person living a more or less standard life in a civilized society. There will be inevitable repetitions of my statements in the current book, but with details and summarization in one procedure. There should be adjuncts that a person can implement in everyday practice while understanding the principles of rational dental hygiene. What works for one person might not work for another. The most important thing is to customize a consistent routine.

Daily dental hygiene activities can be divided into approximately three steps: morning teeth/mouth cleaning and bedtime teeth/mouth care finalization, with teeth/mouth cleaning after food intake. The latter is the main step.

Some comments will accompany the diagram.

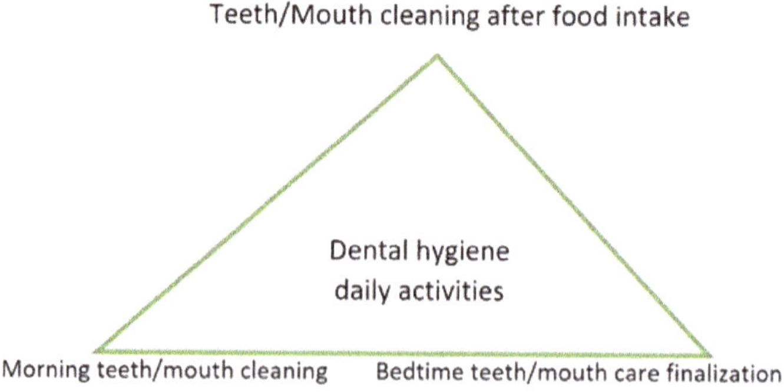

Morning teeth and mouth cleaning include rinsing with water or cosmetic mouthwash. It is a morning "shower." The body would forgive if you skipped it for some reason, but the mouth is less reluctant to accept excuses.

With or without toothbrushing, this activity removes hydrogen sulfide and methyl mercaptan products, the result of microbiota metabolism, including acidic content and gas-emitting bacteria, on the tongue and below the gum line. Cosmetic mouthwash can mask bad breath (halitosis), but water-intensive rinsing is best.

Teeth/mouth cleaning after every food intake is an unrealistic, unachievable goal, but it is in the background of my vision of personal dental hygiene principles. It should be declared and, in whole or in elements of it, implemented. Meanwhile, make it on every occasion, including refraining from mouth "contamination" between regular meals. Eventually, an empty mouth might be the norm.

Bedtime, whenever it occurs, is an opportunity to leave the mouth free from food for a particular time to give the microbiota to settle its ecological relationship. On the one hand, this means a final cleaning following all parts of the procedure, which a person established but had not been implemented during the day for some reason. On the other hand, it is an occasion to use some recommendations for applications that require time for the desired effect reaction. There could be a special need for dentures or flossing under bridges.

A parenthetical suggestion

Food is swallowed, and the acid-containing swallowed soda drink's gas is gone with breath. But remnants of food remain. Permanent on the teeth in the mouth, bacteria inhabitants immediately start their nefarious activities, producing lactic acid that also starts its undesirable chemical reaction at the weak, prone to damage spaces at the teeth.

At the nearest appropriate time, it would not be a bad idea to take out a portable toothbrush and clean your teeth with toothpaste after consuming a delicious French fry or similar starch product, of course, when a pleasant aftertaste is gone. You could also use a portable interdental brush.

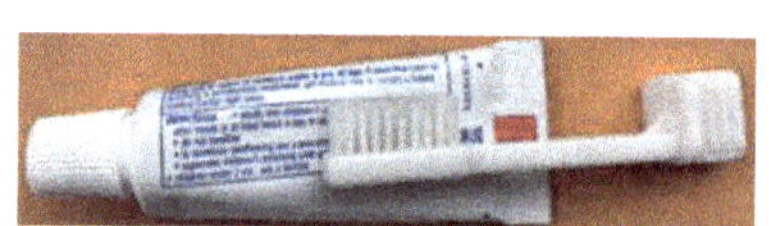
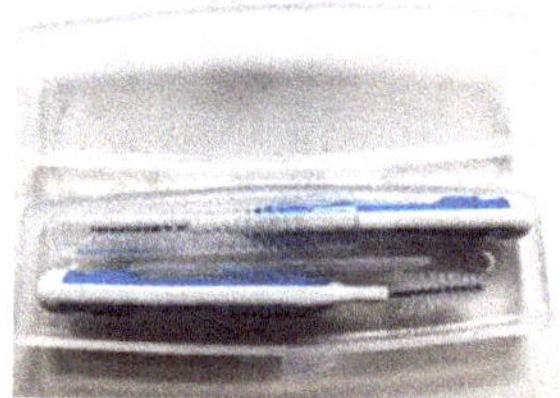

Or just rinse the mouth.

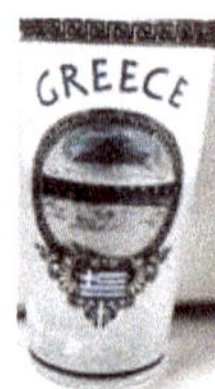

As probably the ancient Greek god of medicine Asclepius' daughter, Hygeia, would suggest.

Standard dental hygiene procedure sequence

The diagram below represents the sequence of actions in this 100-year-long established dental hygiene procedure. I refrain from calling this section an optimal pattern, although I think it is. The sequence of actions should become an automatic routine.

The procedures' descriptions might look like those discussed before, but this repetition, with some details added, serves the purpose of summarization.

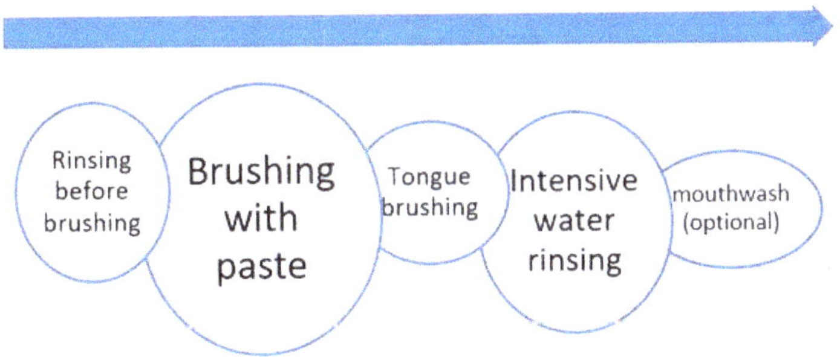

Rinsing before brushing

Rinsing with water or with paste from the tube before brushing removes pieces of food leftovers, especially minute crumbs, to prevent them from reaching subgingival space by accidentally unfortunate brush' bristles movements. If some minute fragments get into the many times mentioned gingival sulcus, the crumb becomes trapped for the microorganism's metabolism consumption. The tongue instead of a brush distributes the paste. The entire mouth should be filled with water. For optimal and desirable final swishing with a favorable mouthwash, start with sipping the foam after pouring warm water into the cup of the mouthwash to reach as many taste receptors of the tongue and mouth as possible; more on pages. 158-164.

However, most dentist usually recommend to start with flossing. This is a disputable issue.

Brushing with paste

Rinsing with paste is also used and reasonable due to foamy condition, but the toothbrushing with paste in the main procedure. Its course follows a scheme determined by tooth design in the alveolar arch. This scheme was mentioned in the *Brushing* section but will be offered here in more detail.

A soft brush and paste provide a thin layer on the bristles. The thinner the layer, the better because otherwise, a thick paste layer would prevent the bristles from reaching every tooth crevice, especially the interdental space. The goal is to leave no tooth behind.

The quality of the paste is also determined by its ability to form such a thin layer after being squeezed from the tube. A thick knob-like squeeze would provide an unequal paste distribution among teeth. As usual, I do not mention any brand.

It is reasonable to cover the entire teeth surface with the paste and wait a few seconds before working with separate groups of teeth just for the "soaking," like in a washer. Paste ingredients move fast into targeting surfaces because it is an osmotic process that requires time to create foam. The foam formation in toothpaste is a coaction of ingredients' surfactant properties, air entrapment, viscosity, and hydration followed by mechanical agitation (more details about foam formation are also *in Appendices* of this book, pages 143-149).

Tongue cleaning

After teeth are done, the tongue's cleaning, actually brushing, turn comes. The necessity of doing this is now common knowledge. It can be done once a day. .First, clean the brush from the paste after cleaning the teeth. The tongue and the gut do not need additional mouth bacteria to its microbiota population.

Placing the additional paste on the brush is unnecessary, but it would not hurt just a thin layer. The brush is placed as deep as possible without initiating a vomiting reflex (emesis). The latter is an important guard from the tongue, and bacterial cleaning debris reaches the gut.

The brush makes energetic strokes move from the roof of the tongue to the tip. The brush's movement should be in one direction along the relatively deep median sulcus of the tongue with the brush's mild pressure on the sulcus. The tongue has a delicate structure (the description in the Anatomy section). The brush's pressure is minimal at the tip to preserve important taste receptors for their sensitive function duties. In the same way, both side areas of the tongue should be preserved from the brush's rough frictions for the same reasons.

Using a different brush for tongue cleaning would not be a bad idea. The brush should have slightly elevated bristles on the upper part.

Water rinsing

Intensive water rinsing is the final, most crucial part of the toothbrushing procedure. In this regard, the foamy paste quality is essential. Vigorous switching creates a foamy environment in the mouth that provides effective cleaning. As mentioned, it is a process similar to a washer cycle or even laundry with some differences Following this analogy, I would suggest some details in rinsing after paste brushing as the final accord that, in my view, determines the result.

The initial amount of water should be minimal (15-30 ml, a half or whole drink). It is like a soaking process in a washer. In contrast with the rigid washer's corpus, the mouth has buccal muscles whose swishing movements can make better contact with paste to generate a foamy content where paste's ingredients, like detergent in a washer, are in closer contact with water. It would be similar to what in chemistry is called the emulsification process.

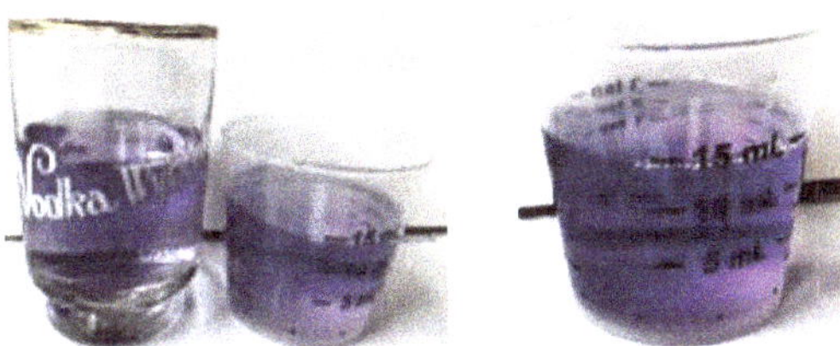

Again, just for orientation.

The word "initial" was included on purpose because the amount of rinsing water should be increased during the next "rinsing sessions." The ultimate goal is to make sure every remnant of food, biofilm, and other debris is "scraped off" from the surfaces of the teeth and mouth alley, especially in the gingival sulcus.

How many? At least three, but more, would be better. Actually, n + 1, when 1 is an additional to your desire to finish. It depends on a person's determination, time allocation, and mood in this situation. We don't live for rinsing our mouths.

An additional detail is the rationality of minimal water in the mouth during initial rinsing. Actually, this applies to every mouth rinse and swish.

The goal is to "peel off" and dislodge residual particles from the interdental space and the gum's gingival sulcus more effectively. The buccal muscles are very powerful; one of them, the masseter muscle, is the most powerful in the body. However, it operates in a limited space in the mouth. It is good for chewing, but it is not designed for swishing during rinsing after tooth brushing.

Minimal water provides more space for vigorous muscle contractions. Intensive swishing generates mechanical vibrations and a temporary vacuum in the local teeth space that extracts tiny remnants after cleaning. A mathematician would describe this using some formulas where perhaps vibrations and vacuum would be included, but we do not go in this math direction.

Mouthwash

Mouthwash products might be considered the final step in tooth brushing. They are optional, depending on individual preferences. If the tooth brushing procedure has been done carefully, the taste in the mouth matters more than finalizing the cleaning process. Cosmetic mouthwashes—or, as I prefer to call them, comfort mouthwashes—should be used just as a reward after the hardship of toothbrushing. For sure, mouthwashes have many pleasant ingredients

The minimal sip of liquid is optimal during toothbrushing. We do not irrigate the mouth but rather try to extract "dirt" from all the ins and outs of the tooth areas.

Mouthwashes are different. Cosmetic comfort mouthwash aims to "please" the areas of the mouth where taste receptors are located, including the taste buds on the top of the tongue at the back. The entire mouth (space) should be filled. In this regard, I would suggest as a final action to place a little (15-20 ml) mouthwash in a cup and pour a stream of preferably warm water to create bubble content, which works more effectively to deliver all ingredients included in the mouthwash.

Some dilution of the mouthwash makes it less irritable, which is reasonable for some mouthwash, more swishing times, and eventually saves money. Some elaboration on mouthwash foam formation is placed in the *Appendices, pages 158-164).* They would bring more understanding to the procedure.

At the end of the prophylactic personal dental hygiene procedures, an example of a situation is placed when they become at the border close to therapeutic.

Suppose a tooth or teeth are unstable (shaky) in the jaw socket. In that case, the personal dental hygiene procedure requires outer support from both sides during brushing, as well as intensive rinsing, including foamy mouthwash.

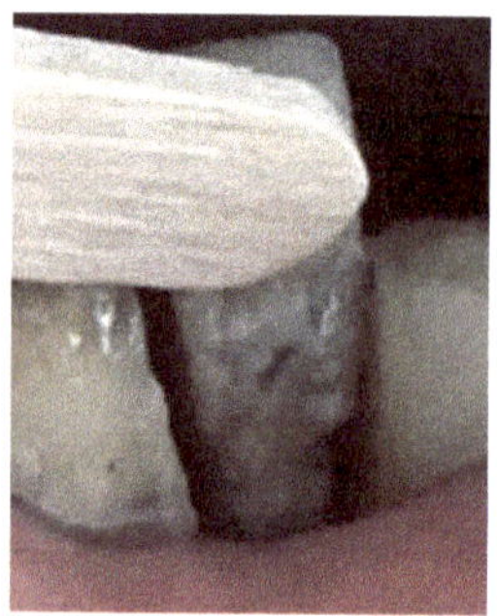

A wooden tongue depressor/tongue blades supports two teeth, but it could be a different method, such as a sponge.

PerioGard should be used with a dentist's advice and prescription. I would add to the PerioGard descriptions on pages 104-105 of the current book some recommendations to use this medication only after a meal without any attempt of spitting it out, being afraid if part or the entire amount is swallowed. The surface of the stomach is so large, and its content is incomparable with the 15 ml, which is a large spoon doze of PerioGard. Swallowing would not be damaging, but the lingering effect of the medication could be beneficial.

Flossing/Interdental cleaning is crucial in this case. I suggest bendable interdental brushes (page 92). These brushes can be used for final cleaning the mouth around the mouth.

 After the procedure, the brushes should be intensively rinsed under running water stream.

Example of personal everyday dental care

A middle age woman Linda X. shared with me her everyday dental care practice. Her teeth are in excellent conditions. He has for some reason three teeth upper Jaw bridge. According to her statement, she does this procedure after every meal intake. She is chewing a gum between them. This was her explanation of refusing any suggested food, agreeing only for water.

The content in her purse related to her dental hygiene routine. The brand names are intentionally omitted to avoid any advertising.

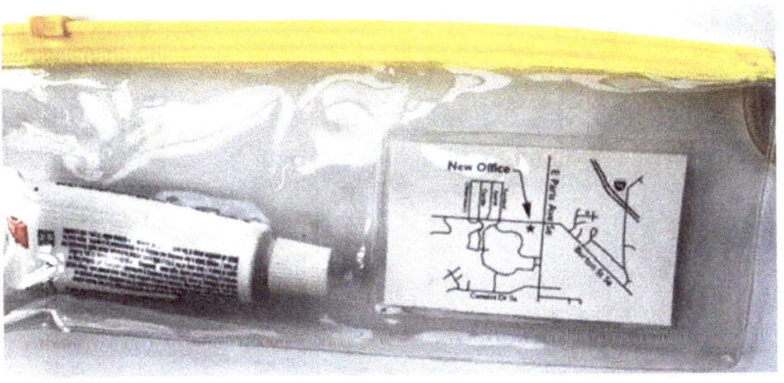

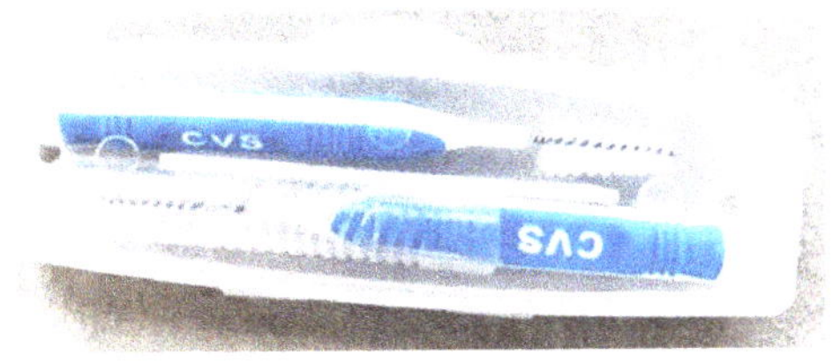

First- picks floss.

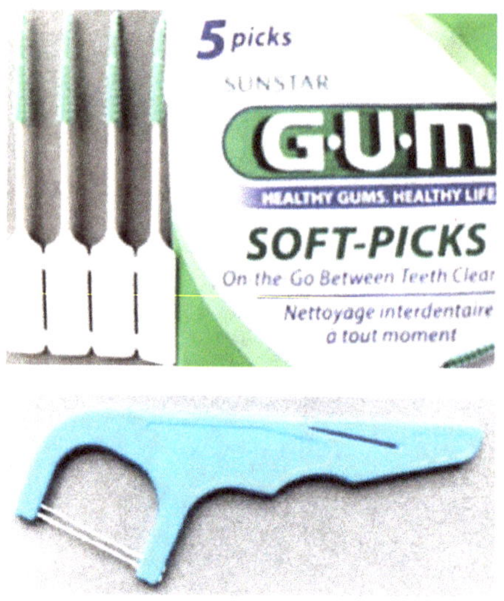

Second -deep clean with a floss tread.

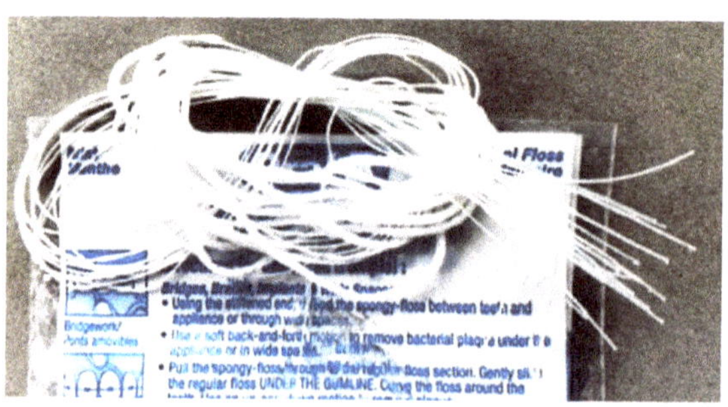

Third dental bridge clean with a thread looking in a portable mirror.

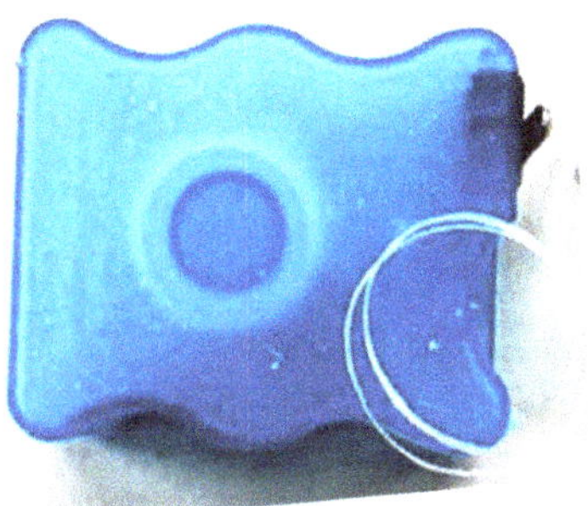

The mirror is also with a tongue scraper in a portable box

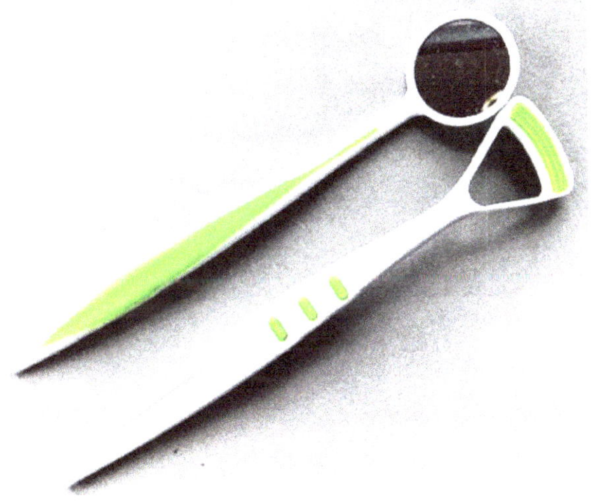

Fourth-portable tooth brush with paste. Uses both Crest and Colgate. Prefers Colgate. She is brushing vertical from both sides. With a soft brush gums massage.

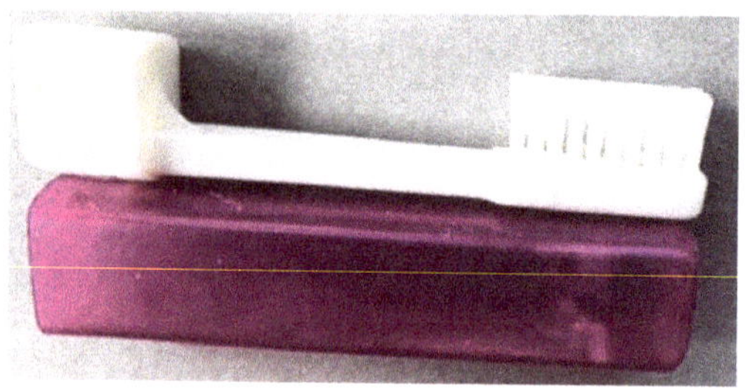

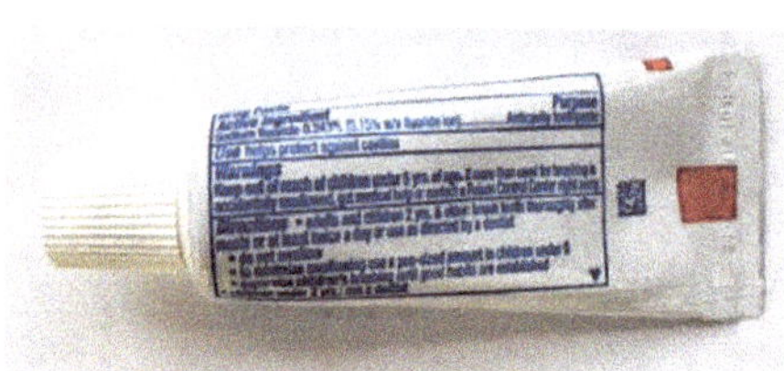

Toothbrush and paste in plastic envelop disposable kit is also in the purse.

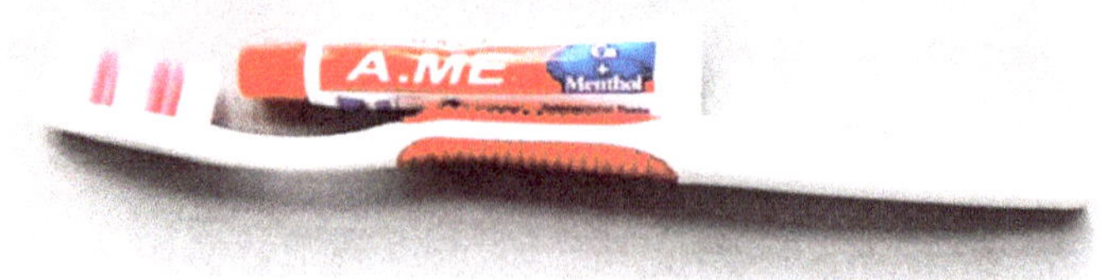

Once a day, at bead time, she is rinsing by using mouthwashes. She is using different brands of them without any preference.

I'm not commenting, except the chewing gum issue. I don't want to argue with American Dental Association's recommendation. In my view, that plague removal is overstatement. The increase saliva output has less acid neutralization ability.

In my believe, chewing gum increases a person's alertness. A good remedy during driving when a person might fall asleep. The current book is finalized by a semiserious entry presented the *Penfield's Homunculus* in support of rinsing the mouth not only as part of dental care. This entry is placed in the *Appendices*.

This section summarizes the previous Methods and Tools Section, which required artificially separating WHAT/WHY, HOW, and WITH to concentrate on the details of each. In reality, this is one process.

In the following section, I'll add a little more "theory" to explain the toothbrushing process, which appears so simple and casual.

Laundry and dishwasher procedures analogy

Just in conclusion of this section, I want to make cloth laundry in a washer as an analogy to teeth brushing action. Actually, laundry follows the same principle as doing dishes.

The shelves in stores of laundry or dishwasher product variants are overwhelming, but for me, as the author of this book, the shelves about dental hygiene in libraries and not bookstores are not intimidating, to my surprise. Few books are predominantly for kids.

Although gentle gum is apparently different from a cowboy's jeans or grime on the plates the cleaning principle is very similar, with all due respect for the sacred toothbrushing ritual.

Laundry washer

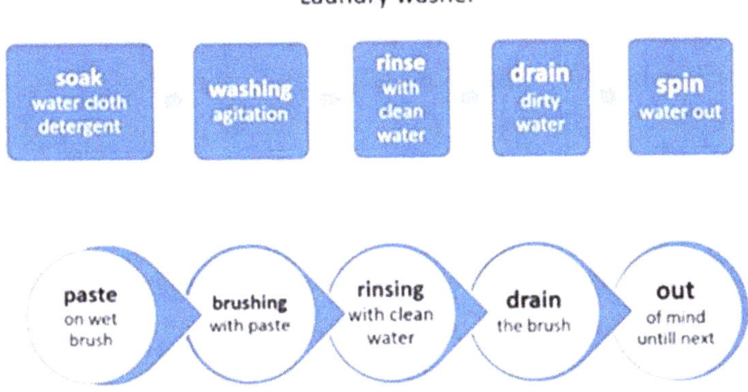

Teeth brushing

While all three cleaning components, chemical, mechanical, and thermal, are apparent in the laundry washer, they are less visible and compressed in tooth brushing.

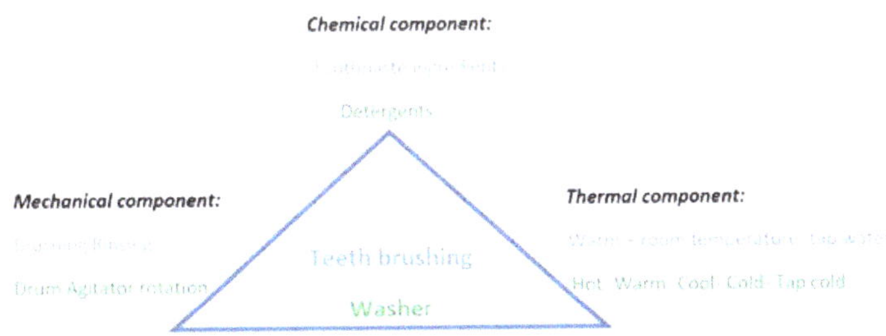

The experience collected by the washer industry should not be ignored because the outcome can be verified, while the result of brushing teeth is more of a hope. A mixture of soap (a surfactant with a low surface tension) and water with a high surface tension generates foam. In a washer, foam extends the surface of detergents' contact with fibers by entering every fabric fiber. The same is true during tooth brushing. For more about the physics of surface tension, see pages 158-164.

A similar process is valid for foamy toothpaste. Foam facilitates surfactant spread. An agitator or impeller in a washer's design is identical to the toothbrush used for different teeth or cleaning situations. Both can change the temperatures of actions and switch the intensity, never mind that the brush's movements are just mechanical parts of the actions. These factors work together to create the foamy texture that aids the distribution of toothpaste during brushing. In principle, there is no difference with washing hands by creating a foamy substance that removes dirt.

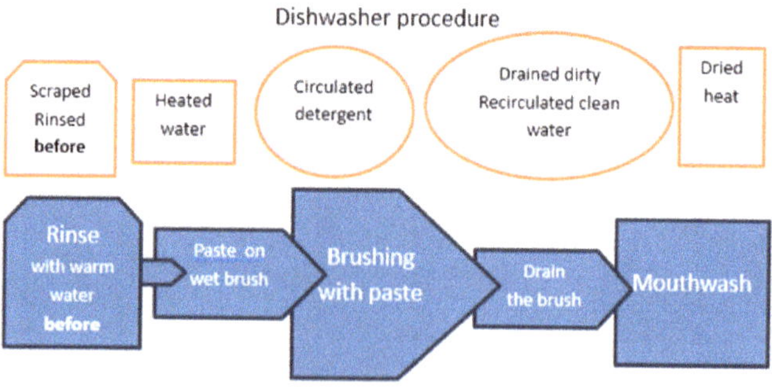

Teeth brushing

Epilogue

This is the general scheme with all deviations determined by a person's particular circumstances and preferences.

As a pathology practitioner, my view of personal dental hygiene, in general, tends to follow an established pattern. I emphasize cleaning the teeth and their mouths home from remnants of food by housekeeping, thus leaving the microbial population to use its own devices to live under something closely resembling a hungry diet. Rinsing is, in my view, the main procedure. Other actions, such as tooth brushing and flossing, are preliminary actions for this final accord. My main premise is sanitation rather than disinfection, as Hygiea Goodness probably had in mind.

Dental hygiene is a part of modern life. It became a necessity determined by civilization's achievements, such as prolonged life expectancy and variegated lifestyles, including dietary diversity. By following the requirements and techniques of personal dental hygiene, the ritual should not override common sense.

Apology for

    boring theory materials

        adherence to details

            repeating many times my main premises

                placing travesty statements.

Appendices

The current book disseminates parenthetical remarks.
Perhaps the entries in the *Appendices* can also be considered
parenthetical to the personal dental hygiene subject.

Remark on dental bridges' longevity

The following remark regarding dental bridges' longevity is
neither a scientific study nor a dental professional
recommendation but rather an invitation to discourse about
one of the humans' achievements in life improvement:
dental bridges. It is more a consideration of a layperson in
dentistry who happens to be a pathology practitioner with
some superficial knowledge of physics that determines a
dental bridge as a mechanical construction in the living
organism's body.

This is why these remarks use both jaw anatomical data and
a regular across-a-river bridge analogy. They consider how
mechanical construction interacts with the product of
millions of years of development, which will concord with the
current book's evolutionary gist. As far as I am aware, the
remarks are focused on assumptions that are not discussed
in the literature. Perhaps they might contribute to dental
bridge longevity practice.

Some basics about dental bridges

A dental bridge sits atop the gums and anchors to a crown on its neighboring teeth. A dental bridge is also called a fixed partial denture [FPD] or fixed dental prosthesis [FDP]). It is an orthopedic structure consisting of crowns combined into a single line. Perhaps a dental prosthesis would be more appropriate to call, especially in science literature, but the bridge is the established term that brings some visualization to the construction.

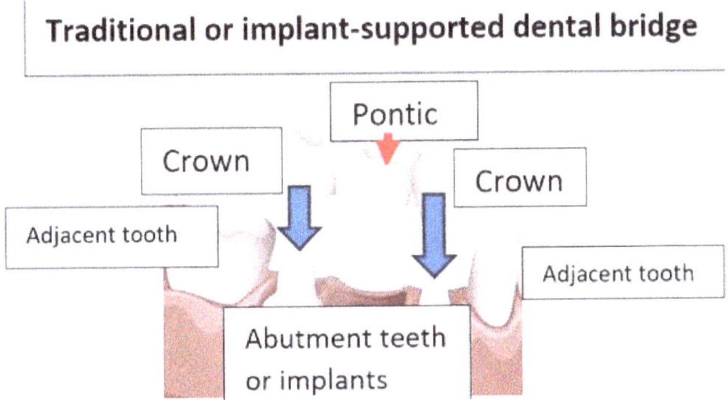

Dental professionals refer to artificial teeth as pontics that fill in the gap of missing teeth. They are anchored to a tooth next to the abutment teeth or a dental implant.

The two outermost crowns have a cavity to be fixed on supports serving as fastening elements. Medium crowns replace 1 to 4 lost dental units and have a one-piece design while leaving space above the gum. The number of replaced teeth depends on concrete dental situations, but the anterior teeth can be for one more replaced unit than chewing teeth.

Traditional Dental Bridge

The traditional fixed bridge, which includes a crown on either side of the pontic/s, is the most popular type. It can be used when a person has natural teeth on either side of the gap between teeth. It is a one-piece bridge made of metal-ceramic or ceramic. The main disadvantage of a traditional bridge is the need to grind down the enamel and some dentin from the abutment teeth to make space for the bridge's two crowns.

Implant-Supported Bridge

An implant-supported bridge requires surgery to place the implants in the jawbone, followed by a period of up to six months that allows the implant to integrate with the jawbone before an implant-supported bridge before mounting the new crown and bridge.

Other types of dental bridges:

Cantilever bridge when there is only one anchor tooth to support the denture. This single-tooth bridge is used when two teeth are missing in a row but is not recommended for use on the third and second molars, where too much bite force may be applied to the abutment tooth or abutment. *Maryland* bridge, which does not require preliminary grinding of the enamel of the abutment teeth due to the attachment with side plates. The construction is used on the front teeth when adjacent teeth are still stable. Only traditional and implant-supported will be discussed

Dental bridges longevity

Theoretically, dental bridges, especially implant-supported ones, can last to the end of a person's life. However, there is no time to confirm this assumption, especially for implant-supported bridges/prostheses. Below is some data from the literature that I could extract.

 "The average dental bridge lasts between five and seven years. With proper care, some bridges can last more than a decade." states most commercial Internet sources.

 Advances in dental bridge materials and methods are likely to make them even more durable in the future. Zaninovich M, Petrucci C. Same day implant bridge for full-arch implant fixed rehabilitation. *J Esthet Restor Dent*. 2019;31(3):190-198. doi:10.1111/jerd.12449.

An example of a bridge longevity

Although a single example does not have credible significance, it may make sense to present it, especially for the following assumption at the end of the current entry. Allegedly, one apple fell on Isaak Newton's head, leading to Newton's law of gravitation discovery.

A traditional metal-ceramic on both sides dental bridge (three units - pontics upper- and four-units- pontics) lower jaws), which lasts 32 years, is on the panoramic roentgenograms (X-ray), and the lower and upper jaw bridges abutment teeth X-rays on the next two pages.

Full-mouth panoramic X-ray. Upper and lower jaw four metal ceramic bridges. Year 2000 X-ray

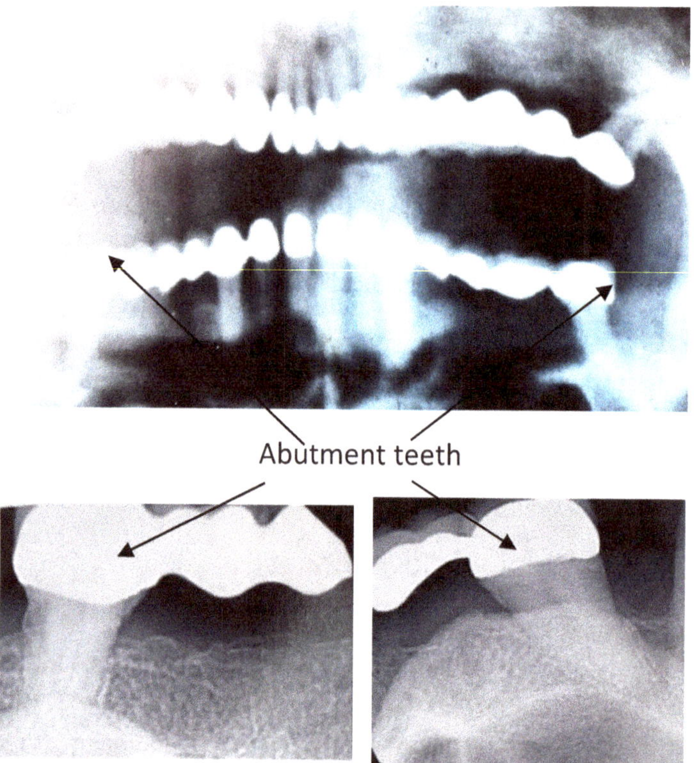

Year 2009 X-ray

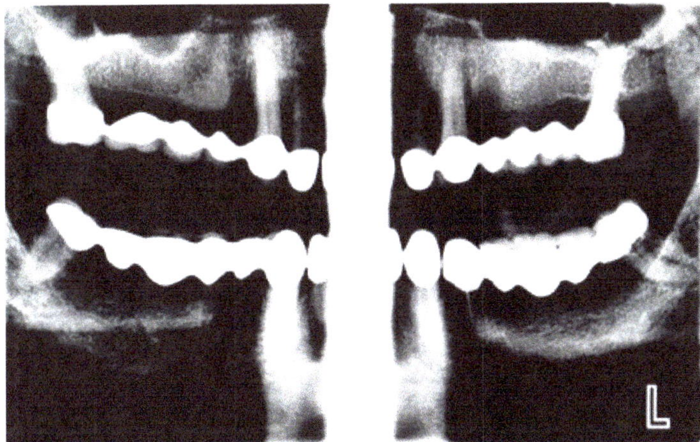

Panoramic X-ray of the traditional metal ceramic bridge.

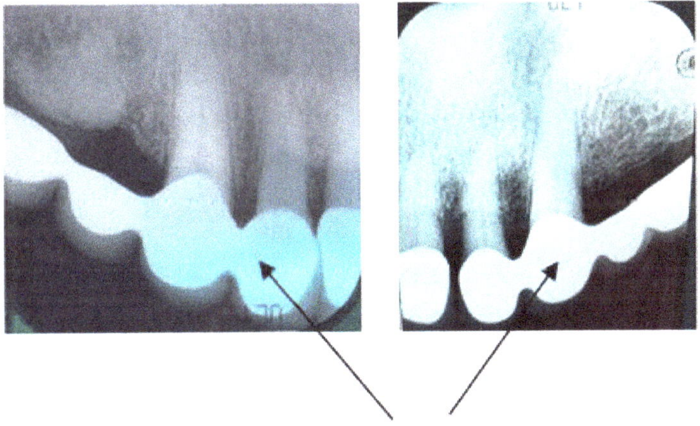

Two abutment teeth (upper jaw)

Two abutment teeth make the bridge construction stronger.

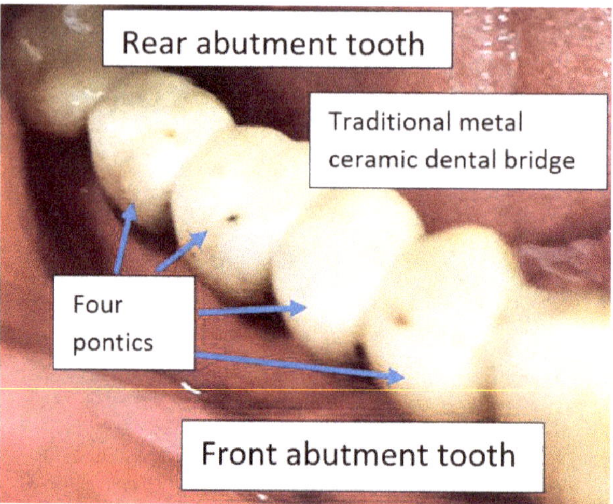

Lower (mandible) jaw traditional metal ceramic bridge (year 2024).

Besides personal dental hygiene procedures at that time (of 90th), the dentist advised the carrier of the bridge some details of food consumption. No special diet, except too much as cracking nuts or similar hard products. Cracker and rusk of any hardness are appropriate, but better on the middle of the bridge. However, chewing simultaneously hard and soft food should be avoided. For example, in the case of a toasted bagel, when the outer part becomes hard, but the internal remains soft, biting and chewing involving the bridge/s and adjacent tooth would be inappropriate.

Why? The regular bridge analogy and considerations presented in the section below will try to prepare to answer this question as an assumption.

Jaw and dental bridge: host and guest

A dental bridge is a kind of prosthesis that, as an intruder in the person's living body, permanently contacts with it, changing the conditions of the place of the intrusion. The famous phrase *In Rome does what the Romans* do not work in this situation.

A reminder from the anatomic part of this book (pages 17-18). The periodontal ligament (PDL) between two teeth, besides other functions in tooth movement, is involved in adjusting to the food's firmness. Otherwise, the tooth would be prone to crashes. In other words, the tooth is held in the socket, which acts as a car's shock absorber.

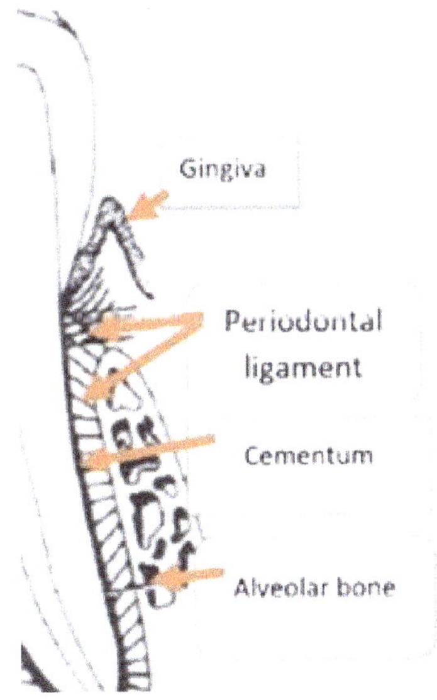

Periodontal ligament (PDL) diagram.

In the case of a traditional dental bridge, most of the abutment teeth PDL are lost during grinding down the enamel and some dentin.

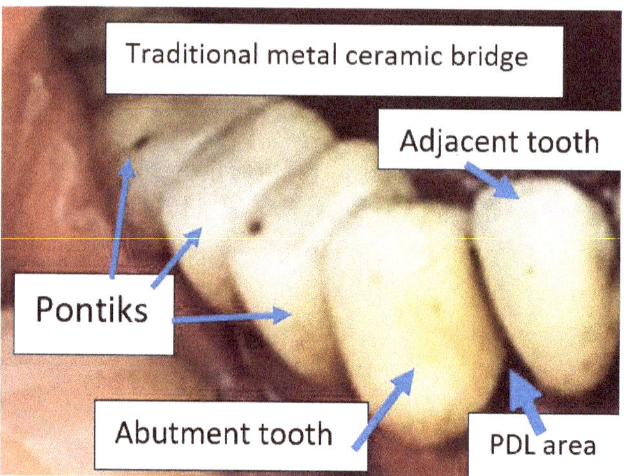

Lower jaw front part of the dental bridge.

In the case of an implant-supported bridge, when the goal is for the implant and jawbone to fuse (Osseo integrated), the PDL cannot be formed during bone growth around the implant. The bone formed around the implant is predominantly cancellous with cortical elements.

As a result, PDL works only from one side of the carried bridge abutment pillar tooth, while it is not balanced by the same distribution of force at the adjacent tooth. There is also the absence of micro-mobility of teeth (as separate independent elements) because the bridge is a fixed, monolithic structure.

This entry is about dental bridges longetivity. Let's follow the fate of already mentioned (pages 137-139) five teeth traditional bridge.

 It was plced in the jaw of now 86 year old man 34 years ago. (See the 2000, 2019 and 2025 x-rays).

There is evidence of bone resorption under one of the abuntment teeth. On the x-rays, the arrows point the resorbtion area at the front teeth of the left lower jaw.

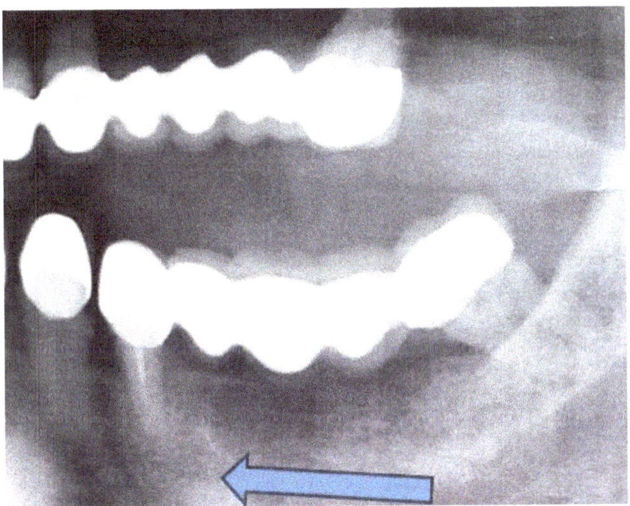

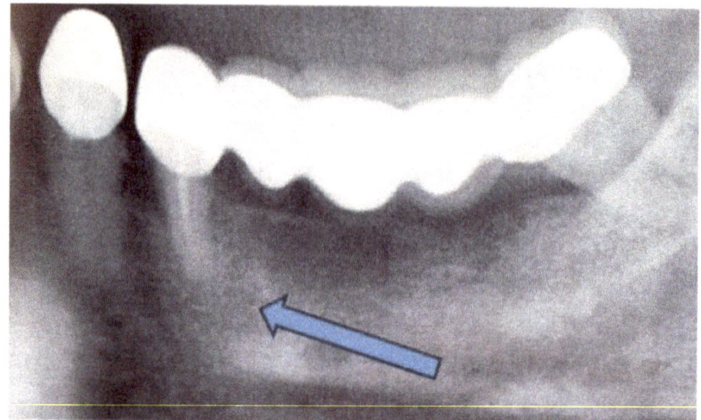

This causes some instability, moving "fluctuation" of the bridge. that requires minimal participation in chewing by the left side of the mouth and more careful dental hygiene procedure, including flossing and rinsing and changes in the mode of the procedure. Adjustments to everyday dental hygiene procedure are determined by the gap between the abutment's crown and the gum.

Complete or partial of it would be reasonable after every meal, especially when small crumbs of food are generated. The procedure should start with rinsing. A soft brush with first horizontal and then vertical brushing would be correct.

.

Dental bridge and a regular bridge analogy

A transportation bridge ends up with ground or other surface connection as a dental bridge with adjacent teeth area.

Below is a diagram of a regular bridge structure's essential supporting part. The focus is on the bridge abutment, the elements at the ends of a bridge, which provide support by absorbing the forces placed on the bridge, preventing the earth under the approach to the bridge from moving.

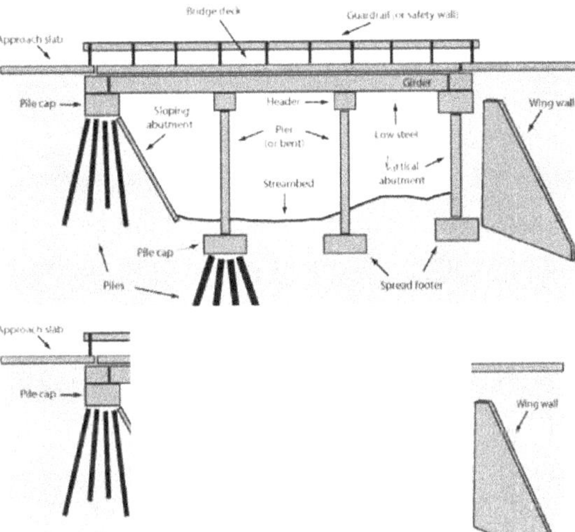

The diagram of the essential parts of a bridge structure. (Adapted with modification from *CivilArcCivil Engineering, Architecture & Design*).

Chewing generates a significant force applied on a relatively small surface of the dental unit. The abutment teeth or an implant screw would be an analogy.

A bridge's foundation (or base) connects the structure to the earth and transfers loads to the ground below. The diagram shows that the foundation abutment has additional construction support as a sloping abutment and wing wall. The pile cap supports the approach slab.

An assumption on dental bridge longevity

A regular transportation bridge and a dental bridge encounter the same circumstance when a loaded cargo train/car and a piece of unequal-consistency food reach the end of the construction. However, the pressure of the force of weight is different in these two parts of the construction.

 The enhanced foundation (or base) prepares the transportation bridge to resist the difference. The jaw with a dental bridge is deprived of such a compensation mechanism due to a one-sided periodontal ligament (traditional dental bridge) or the absence of the latter (implant-supported dental bridge).

The dental bridge becomes like a car with malfunctioning shock. Eventually, due to many conditions in the jaw (periodontitis, atrophy of the jawbone at the bridge site by uneven loading, etc.), the stability of the dental construction becomes impaired, especially for older bridge carriers. Moreover, the area of abutment and adjacent teeth becomes more vulnerable and prone to local complications. This is the argument for stricter adherence to principles of personal dental hygiene by carefully following the procedures, including interdental cleaning.

In both dental and regular transportation bridges, the basic physics laws of gravitation, all three Newton's laws can be applied, and even Archimedes-the law of the lever, but the most relevant would-be Hooke's law of elasticity. Regular bridge builders can calculate the construction using their math apparatus, while in the case of a dental bridge, we have to deal with the summarization of their effect.

The presented assumption explains the dentist's rationale for avoiding unequal hard/soft food consistency to maintain a dental bridge's longevity. Although dentists do not recommend nuts and other hard food consumption, in my understanding, the hardness does not matter substantially due to the quality of modern materials when the hard component of food (nut, for example)) is masticated in the center of a bridge. The main challenges are at the ends of the bridge.

However, it is apparently difficult to manage food's location during chewing; avoiding such challenges would be rational. Of course, there could be numerous individual and food exclusions.

 The assumption is open for discussion. Different opinions would definitely benefit the increasing number of dental bridge carriers.

Reflections on halitosis and dental hygiene

Bad breath (halitosis, oral malodor) might be a symptom of periodontitis or sometimes serious diseases, which I do not want to mention avoiding iatrogenic disease (iatros -Ancient Greek word for a doctor) among people prone to phobias.

There is a condition that is defined as delusional halitosis or imaginary halitosis when people believe that their breath odor is a social nuance without any objective proof. Delusional halitosis occurs not so rarely. Halitosis is a serious psychosomatic problem, and manufacturers of mouthwashes and other dental hygiene products are not completely innocent. Moreover, bad breath is personal and cultural, with many nuances, including individual smells. Modern society has become too sensitive, a "sniffing society."

I want to reflect on just the smell emanating from a person's mouth, which is better to call unpleasant for its recipient, without stepping on psychology-related territories. I want to focus on the smell that is physiologically generated by the tongue's microbiota metabolism. To narrow the subject as part of oral/dental hygiene. As with everything in this book, this reflection is my view on the subject. I had an accident experience when hydrogen sulfide (H_2S) escaped from the synthesis apparatus and required evacuation from the building due to the real intolerable smell.

 It is a consensus that intraoral conditions are the cause of halitosis in 80-85% due to periodontal infections (Halitosis: Current concepts on etiology, diagnosis, and management (Eur J Dent. 2016 10(2): 292–300). The tongue can be held responsible for keeping onto food particles and plaques of bacteria colonies between papillae that produce Volatile Sulfur Compounds (VSCs). They include hydrogen sulfide (H_2S), methyl mercaptan, and dimethyl sulfide, with a sharp, unpleasant, irritating odor.

Human evolution, which lasted millions of years, ended with the formation on the tongue dorsum's back of an area populated with a group of bacteria (anaerobic, gram-negative) with proteolytic activity that generates VSCs. Why are these groups of bacteria concentrated in the back of the tongue, along with most of the taste buds and the mouth lymphatic tissue ring? This is the area where the body finally encounters the outside environment, one of the significant defense lines of the gut and lungs.

This superficial consideration is presented to justify my respect for evolutionary-developed biological structures, in this case, the tongue microbiota. It needs defense from assault by too vigorous oral/dental hygiene activity.

Cleaning from excesses of microbiota hyperproduction is rational because modern life is challenging the evolutionary-established oral cavity homeostasis. However, any effort to exterminate tongue microflora would be counterproductive. Halitosis is not the target or the goal by itself; oral/dental health is.

Bacteremia and dental hygiene

Introduction

Blood is sterile except in the close-to-death situation of septicemia, sepsis, or exacerbation of infectious endocarditis (*Septica Lenta*). At least, I lived with these postulates until I started reading dental hygiene literature. I was aware of recommendations, even requirements, for prophylactic amoxicillin antibiotics before dental hygienists started to care for people with artificial heart valves. I discovered that bacteremia, the presence of bacteria in the bloodstream, occurs regularly, not only during the hygienist's care but also during standard everyday tooth brushing. Moreover, this bacteremia is linked to the development of infective endocarditis.

Dental bacteremia notion history

An article that stated that the practice of dental extractions led to the entrance of bacteria into the bloodstream was published in 1945. (Bender IB, Pressman RS. *Factors in dental bacteremia. J Am Dent Assoc.* 1945; 32: 836–853). The article was unnoticed at that time.

Five articles were published related to bacteremia as a toothbrushing outcome between 1954 and 1977.
On this subject, an explosion of articles erupted at the beginning of the 21st century.

Different approaches to antibiotic prophylactic

Different and evolving clinical approaches to prophylactic infective endocarditis are based on the pathophysiological definition of bacteremia whose existence after dental procedures is accepted as an indisputable fact. Only its clinical implications are discussed.

The *Circulation* journal published a review article in 2019 of the American Heart Association (AHA) recommendations for antimicrobial prophylaxis for infective endocarditis guidelines evolution since 1955. The AHA abandoned the recommendation of antibiotic prophylaxis based on the lifetime risk of developing infective endocarditis in 2007. The guidelines focused on the greatest risk of infective endocarditis outcomes after some procedures. Among them is dental care.

Professional societies on antibiotic prophylactic

The American Dental Association (ADA), the Infectious Diseases Society of America (IDSA), and the Pediatric Infectious Diseases Society (PIDS)recommended antibiotic prophylaxis in dental procedures but only for patients in high-risk situations, such as those with a prior history of infective endocarditis (IE), a prosthetic heart valve, or Congenital heart abnormalities.

The European Society of Cardiology (ESC), endorsed by the AHA, recommended antibiotic prophylaxis only for high-risk patients of IE and in dental treatments involving manipulation of the periapical region, gingival tissue, or perforation of the oral mucosa.

The British Society for Antimicrobial Chemotherapy (BSAC) recommended covering all bleeding procedures in 1992. The British Cardiac Society and the Royal College of Physicians (BCS/RCP) recommended antibiotic prophylaxis for all dental procedures that might cause bacteremia, as well as those related to heart defects and heart surgery, in 2004.

The British Society for Antimicrobial Chemotherapy (BSAC) recommended in 2006, endorsing the recommendations made in France, antibiotic prophylaxis use only for high-risk patients of BE in cases where these patients were at high risk of death. But in 2008, the National Institute for Health and Clinical Excellence (NICE) in the UK recommended that antibiotic prophylaxis use was no longer needed in dental practice

National and international societies encourage rational approaches to antibiotic prophylaxis for dental procedures by opposing the indiscriminate use of antimicrobial medications.

Some studies concluded that *"there is no scientific evidence demonstrating that antibiotic prophylaxis is effective to prevent infective endocarditis. Moreover, the absence of large-scale clinical trial publications demonstrating the effectiveness of prophylaxis is a fact. For this reason, these guidelines have been questioned"* (Oliver et al. Antibiotics for the prophylaxis of bacterial endocarditis in dentistry. Cochrane Database Syst Rev. 2008;4:CD003813.).

Some references

Kinane DF et al. Bacteremia following periodontal procedures. J Clin Periodontol. 2005; 32:708-713.

Bacteremia and Oral Health. Maintaining oral health may be more effective than antibiotic prophylaxis in reducing the risk of bacteremia. Dimensions on dental hygiene. Gen Benoit, et al .2012. A quote: "Among those at elevated risk of BAC (Bacteremia), benign activities such as **toothbrushing, flossing**, using **toothpick**s or **oral irrigating devices**, and **chewing can cause BAC.**"

Incidence of bacteremia after chewing, tooth brushing, and scaling in individuals with periodontal inflammation. Forner Lone et al., Periodontology 2006.

Bacteremia due to dental flossing. Crasta Kenneth et al. J Clin Periodontology.2009 Apr;36(4):323-32.

Incidence and magnitude of bacteremia caused by **flossing** and by **scaling** and **root planning**. William Zhang et al. Journal of Clinical Periodontology. 2013 Jan;40(1):41-52.

Methodology aspect

The article *Bacteremia Associated with Toothbrushing and Dental Extraction* (Peter B. Lockhart, et al. Circulation. 2008; 117:3118–3125) can be interesting from the methodology aspect of how studies on bacteremia are conducted. The author worked on the subject since the late 1980s. He published many articles and was cited in every publication on bacteremia.

Excerpts from the article's *Material and methods*:

For bacterial isolation and Identification, blood samples were cultured in BACTEC Plus Aerobic/F and LYTIC/10 Anaerobic/F, and the 16S ribosomal RNA (rRNA) sequencing method was used for bacterial identification. Bacterial lysates were used as templates in polymerase chain reaction with 16S rRNA universal primers according to standard protocols. Sensitive, real-time, quantitative polymerase chain reaction was used to quantify bacteria....The sensitivity of the method was 25 colony-forming units (CFU) per polymerase chain reaction, which corresponds to 103 to 104 CFU per milliliter of blood.

In my view, the 16S rRNA gene sequence-based bacterial analysis is appropriate in molecular biology science studies, but it is too sensitive in revelation microbial species, which might have diagnostic value with clinical implications. This brings into play vague definitions like associated non-associated bacteria with infective endocarditis. There is no corroborated scientific proof of bacteremia during dental hygiene procedures.

Pathophysiology considerations

Over 700 species of bacteria colonize the human oral cavity, 400 of which were found in the periodontal pocket adjacent to teeth. (Paster BJ, et al. The breadth of bacterial diversity in the human periodontal pocket and other oral sites. Periodontal. 2000. 2006; 42: 80–87.)

Bacteria are not free-floating in the mouth environment; in the different kinds of biofilms, they adhere to the surfaces of the host tissues. Theoretically, they can be detached from the surfaces predominantly by mechanical force during tooth extraction (minimal), tooth brushing (maximal because it is the aim of the procedure), flossing (less than brushing), or chewing (just by accident).

Remnants of bacterial biofilm can sneak into the blood system as a bacteremia phenomenon only when there is a break of continuity or through the lymphatic system. Each of these systems has its defense mechanisms against an intruder.

Immediately after encountering bacteria, a "foreign body", in the reticuloendothelial system, the lymphatic system starts its immunological defense mechanism at the local level with humoral reactions. The final gatekeeper is the lymphoid circle of the mouth, the most developed cellular part, which is the main entrance to the outer world.

Interruption to the continuity of the blood circulation system can occur during mechanical manipulations in the mouth area at the level of the capillary and venule vessels. At the venule level, the thrombi formation immediately starts while bleeding continues from the arteriole-capillary system due to the blood pressure.

This brings me to difficulties in understanding how bacteremia can occur during dental procedures. Even if some remnant of biofilm sneaked into the blood circularity system, diluted in seven liters of blood, and discovered by molecular biology tests, what is the clinical meaning of this? There should be serious preconditions for the smooth endocardium endothelium to incorporate them.

Bacteremia cannot be without a temporal pyrogenic reaction. Sensitive body temperature measurements should reveal this, but I haven't seen any study.

I cannot understand why gastrointestinal or gynecological manipulations with their reach microflora, especially during delivery, are not the sources for bacteremia, never mind after a gangrene amputation surgery. All my experience of thousands of autopsies performed cannot comprehend this.

Antibiotic prophylaxis practice

By the way, the one dose of amoxicillin before dental manipulations imposed on people with heart valve surgery is not only ineffective but contra-productive. It became a dental office ritual that can contribute to drug resistance, making a person vulnerable in front of other occasions of the need to use this antibiotic.

Summary

The clinically significant bacteremia notion during dental hygiene procedures, is exaggerated.

Antibiotic prophylaxis before dental hygiene procedures is counterproductive.

Mouthwash foam formation physics

A foam is a dispersion of gas bubbles in a liquid. In the case of mouthwash, foam is a mass of large and small bubbles formed predominantly on the liquid.

A rationale for using mouthwash this way is that its foamy content reaches more taste receptors, distributing between the smallest papillae of the tongue.

Foam formation

Discussing some details of foam formation when using mouthwash would be reasonable. They would help clarify the procedure.

Foam is a network of air bubbles in thin films. Its formation follows the basic physics law of water's surface tension. A foam bubble is created when the surface tension of water at the surface layer is reduced, allowing gas to mix in.

 A liquid in a thin foam form can reach more targeted surfaces with the chemicals dissolved in it for a specific purpose. The same physics laws work in forming foam in champagne, soft drinks, beer, washing hands, doing dishes, and doing laundry. In dental hygiene, the same can be applied to toothpaste and mouthwash.

It is necessary to mention the difference between foam and froth, for example, in coffee brewing, when the development of bubbles above the liquid surface is more similar to that of cold beverages.

There is also a difference when a mixture of soap and water generates foam. For a comparison with mouthwash foam formation, it would be better to go with beer head, although Coffee Foam (macrofoam) is similar to a froth (micro foam) for a "wet" cappuccino, which is a hot beverage.

The physics and chemistry background of beer head foam formation is the subject of many studies. According to the article The physics and chemistry of beer foam: a review (*Eur Food Res Technol* 249, 3–11 (2023), a stable and appealing foam on beer depends on the balance of foam-positive foaming components (polypeptides, hop bitter acids, metal ions, melanoidins) over foam-negative entities (ethanol, lipids, detergents).

There are studies on foam-stabilizing proteins contributed by malted barley, Lipid Transfer Protein (LTP1), and hordein as forming foam-stabilizing bubbles chemicals. I am not going further with studies that replicate the process in a simulation that solves the Navier–Stokes equation for a mixture of two fluids: liquid beer and CO_2 gas (dol.org/10.1063/PT.6.1.20230307a), as well as with another research. While beer brewers and mouthwash manufacturers will hopefully produce continue studies on optimal components and ingredients, for our goal of optimal use of mouthwashes is more useful the bartenders experience and skills in pouring beer into the glass.

I want to concentrate on performance issues, leaving aside the chemistry of beer brands and ingredients in different types of mouthwash. The bartender's performance is incomparably more complicated and depends on many factors, for example, how clean a glass is for lacing. Issues are generally similar to mouthwash foam generation in dental hygiene procedures.

Inevitably, I have to mention some physics laws to support my foam formation notions. The material below might look boring and too long. It can be omitted, but it is in line with the main premise of the presented book: bringing some high school-level science into such everyday routines as personal dental hygiene. Otherwise, my recommendations would be less understandable.

Foam formation cannot be understood without the physics definition of the surface tension of the liquid. We encounter the phenomenon of surface tension of liquids every day. It is in the background of a drop of water on the end of the dripping faucet or the tap water jet tends to be cylindrical, a steel needle floating on the water's surface, or a water strider can glide on the water's surface.

Surface tension forces act along the surface of a fluid to reduce its area. It's as if the liquid is encased in an elastic film that tends to compress its contents. This allows the substance to retain volume (but not its shape), and this volume is limited to the surface of the liquid. The surface tension of water is much higher than any other known liquid.

The molecular theory of water surface tension, which can be applied to foam formation, views any liquid as a conglomerate of molecules that exert an attractive force on each other. In other words, surface tension occurs because molecules of a liquid attract one another. The potential energy of mutual attraction of liquid molecules is approximately equal to their kinetic energy.

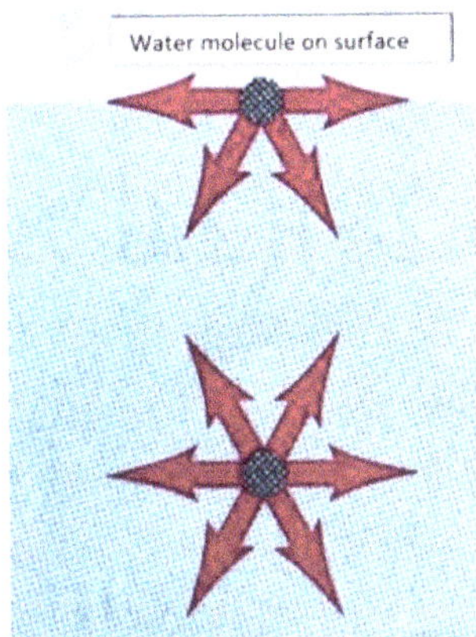

The molecules inside the liquid are in equilibrium because the forces of other molecules act in all directions. The molecule on the surface does not have such equilibrium but still cannot escape due to the presence of molecules below and alongside it. Therefore, a net attractive force downward still compresses the surface layer.

This compression means that liquids minimize their surface area, tending to form spherical droplets representing the minimum surface area for a given volume.

The molecule that is on the surface is affected by the forces of attraction not only from other molecules of the liquid but also from the gas (external environment). The latter is much smaller than the former, so the resultant force of attraction is directed inside the liquid, which helps to hold the molecule on the surface.

Surface tension is a quantity that shows a fluid's tendency to reduce its free surface. The larger the liquid's surface area, the more molecules have excess potential energy, and the greater the surface energy.

 Some force is required to increase a liquid's surface area. Such force can be provided by heat (boiling), sun and wind (evaporation), or chemicals (soaps, detergents, and surfactants). Some energy is required to break the molecules loose from their relatively fixed position in potential energy into kinetic energy with a temporary gaseous phase result, namely foam in our case.

The capillarity phenomenon, where surface tension plays a role in the so-called wetting process, relates to the foam's interaction with the targeted surface. This issue is beyond the foam formation subject.

By the way, a remainder from the laundry washer or dishwasher analogy: Special wetting agents' detergents are often added to water to prevent it from collecting in droplets on any surface. Once in the surface layer of water, the molecules of such reagents noticeably weaken the surface tension forces, so the water does not collect in droplets.

The material above is adapted from various sources, including *Physics: Principles with Applications* by Douglas C. Gialionli, Fifth Edition, 1980, and my high school physics course recollections.

Practical applications of surface tension phenomenon

I want to focus on three factors influencing mouthwash foam formation: the process's agitation, the amount of mouthwash in a glass or plastic cup, and the temperature of the combined liquid (mouthwash + water).

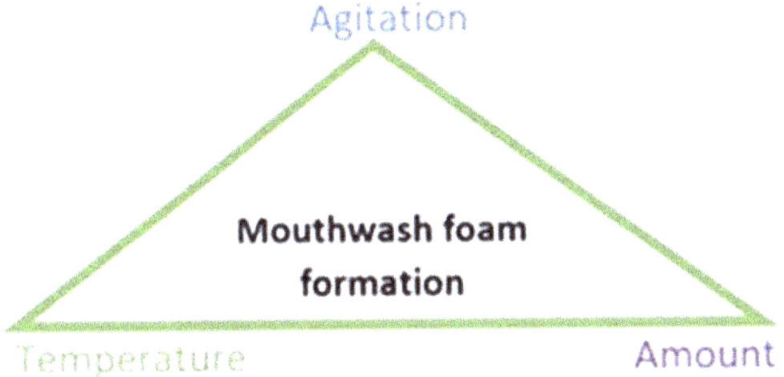

Agitation. Foam formation requires some energy to remove the liquid molecules from their surface because they are held by surface tension. Tap water pouring from a faucet provides such energy by transforming the potential energy into kinetic movement energy of the liquid (water + mouthwash). It is necessary to provide a level of turbulence at the surface and deeper in the liquid.

An analogy would be boiling on heat, water evaporation under the sun, cappuccino brewing, or just pouring beer into a glass. Of course, the content of ingredients is a condition for foam generation of bubble's small size and their sustainability.

The **amount** of mouthwash should be minimal to overcome the liquid's surface tension. The thinner the layer, the less surface tension energy. However, considering the dilution, the amount should be enough to keep the ingredients active for their targeted purpose.

Depending on the time allocated to mouthwash rinsing, I would recommend starting with 5 ml, then 10 ml, and then 15 ml for the most concentrated mouthwash residual effect.

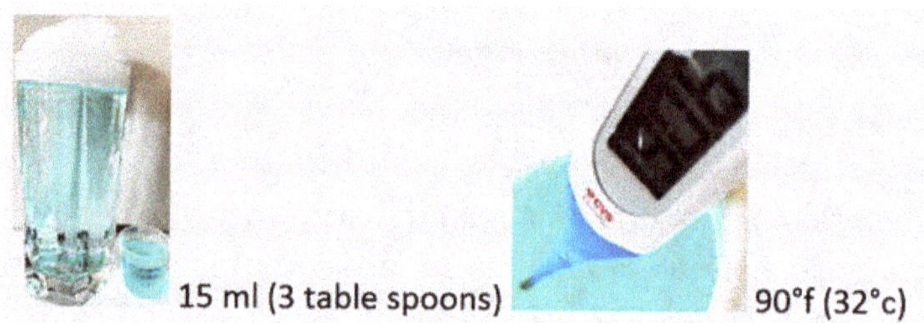

15 ml (3 table spoons)   90°f (32°c)

Of course, **temperature** is a significant parameter. Cold tap water is around 60 F (15.55 C), while room-temperature water is around 78 F (25.55 C). Beers are used between 40 and 50 F. Neither temperature is appropriate for mouthwash foam generation. The optimal tap water temperature should be around 90 F (32 C) to support agitation energy.

Penfield's homunculus and mouth rinsing

Canadian neurosurgeon Wilder Penfield published his famous "motor homunculus" experiments on a diagram in 1940. The diagram shows the area of the cerebral cortex approximately responsible for controlling different parts of the body.

Since 1950, some parts of Penfield's homunculus, which shows the area of the cerebral cortex approximately responsible for the control of different parts of the body, are still being clarified and even disputed today. For example, genitals, which were absent from the original "classic" diagram, have now been located in the cortex below the torso and above the foot. Research is ongoing in this field, even in the 21st century. The mouth and all its attributes, such as lips, tongue, and jaw, remain in the same place.

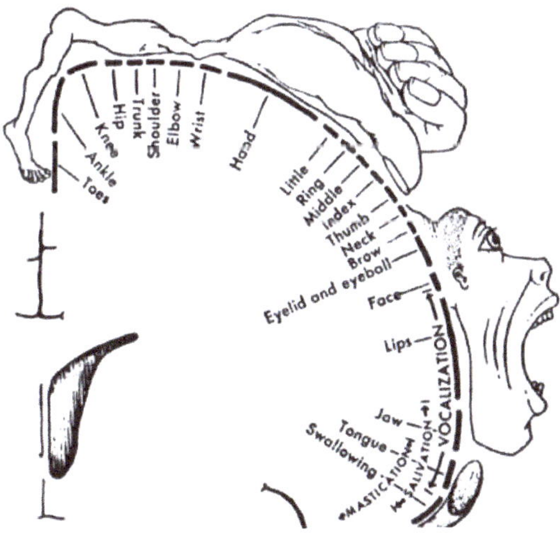

The size of the lips and tongue on Penfield's homunculus map is justifiably connected with vocalization while swallowing and massification are placed inferiorly. The cortical activity is stimulated by vocalization. Refraining from numerous flat jokes on this subject, I want to come closer to the subject of this book, namely, dental hygiene.

Let's silence vocalization by putting some liquid in the mouth for rinsing. From the previous pages of this book, the reader could likely determine that rinsing is my favorite part of dental hygiene procedures. According to Penfield's diagram, I aim to draw attention to the opportunity to stimulate a person's cortex activity by vigorous swishing during rinsing.

As mentioned in the main part of the book, the mouth's muscles are the most powerful in the body, given their short size and ability to contract. During vigorous swishing, most of these muscles are involved. The less liquid in the mouth, the more space the buccal muscles have for swishing, and the more brain-stimulating impulses are sent. Every theoretical assumption requires experimental proof, however. This is the spirit of the suggested book.

Hopefully, Penfield's homunculus will persuade people to rinse their mouths vigorously if they feel drowsy instead of having an extra coffee. The teeth and mouth environment would benefit from these actions. Perhaps some perfect thoughts will come, a person will think more clearly, or a problem will be resolved.

By the way, most business meetings are accompanied by eating and some ritual drinking. Before the digestion starts, that moves intensive blood supply to the digestion area, eating/chewing/drinking actions stimulate the brain alertness.

Perhaps it might be right to finish this essentially boring book about personal dental hygiene routine with the remainder of Penfield's homunculus as my support for rinsing. The latter is my preference for the basic triad: brushing, flossing, and rinsing.

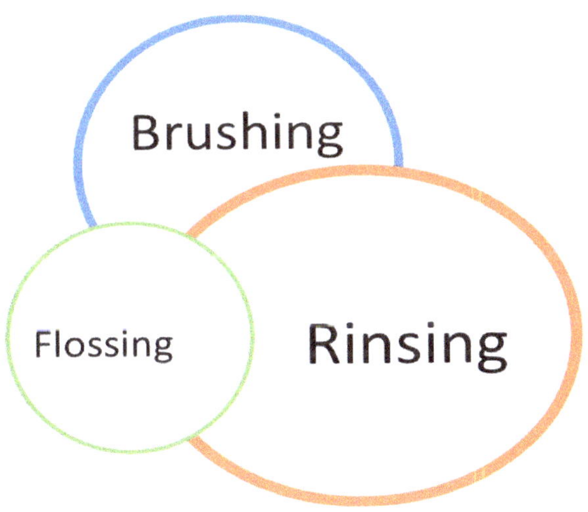

Books on my shelf and Kindle

Lokensgard Thomas Matters of your mouth

Heal your oral microbiome Kindle

Phillips Ellie Mouth care comes clean

Phillips Ellie Kiss your dentist goodbye

Wray David and Alyson Understanding Your Teeth and Mouth

Artemis Nadine Holistic Dental Care: The Complete Guide to Healthy Teeth and Gums

Hoss Kami If Your Mouth Could Talk: An In-Depth Guide to Oral Health and Its Impact on Your Entire Life

Magleby Ben Dr. Ben's Dental Notebook: A Collection of Dental Illustrations, Handouts and Diagrams

Heither the Hygienist The Great Tooth Deception. Revealing the Dark side of Dentistry

Prives Michaell Human Anatomy

Mosby's Comprehensive Review of Dental Hygiene textbook for hygienists

For remarks and comments